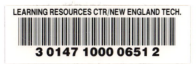

An Atlas of
TRAUMA MANAGEMENT
THE FIRST HOUR

THE ENCYCLOPEDIA OF VISUAL MEDICINE SERIES

An Atlas of
TRAUMA
MANAGEMENT
THE FIRST HOUR

Bridget A. Landon
St. Bartholomew's Hospital
London

P.A. Driscoll
Hope Hospital, Salford

John D. Goodall
St. Mary's Hospital
London

The Parthenon Publishing Group
International Publishers in Medicine, Science & Technology

LONDON   *CASTERTON*   NEW YORK

British Library Cataloguing-in-Publication Data
Landon, Bridget A.
    Atlas of Trauma Management: First Hour. –
(Encyclopedia of Visual Medicine Series)
I. Title   II. Series
617.1
ISBN 1-85070-411-2

Library of Congress Cataloging-in-Publication Data
Landon, Bridget A., 1960–
    An atlas of trauma management: the first hour / Bridget A.
    Landon. Peter Driscoll, John D. Goodall.
       p.   cm. – (The Encyclopedia of visual medicine series)
    Includes index.
    ISBN 1-85070-411-2
    1. Traumatology–Atlases.   2. First aid in illness and injury
    – Atlases.   I. Driscoll, Peter, 1955–   .   II. Goodall,
    John D., 1960–   .   III. Title.   IV. Series.

    RD93.3.L36   1993
    617.1'026'0222–dc20   92-36453
                                                                CIP

Published in the UK and Europe by
The Parthenon Publishing Group Limited
Casterton Hall, Carnforth
Lancs. LA6 2LA

Published in North America by
The Parthenon Publishing Group Inc.
One Blue Hill Plaza
PO Box 1564, Pearl River
New York 10965, USA

Copyright © 1994 Parthenon Publishing Group Ltd

First published 1994

Typeset by AMA Graphics Ltd., Preston
Reproduction by Ryburn Publishing Services, Keele University
Printed and bound in Great Britain by Butler & Tanner Ltd.,
Frome and London

Contents

The Encyclopedia of Visual Medicine Series

Titles currently planned in this series include:

An Atlas of Oncology
An Atlas of Hypertension
An Atlas of Common Diseases
An Atlas of Osteoporosis
An Atlas of the Menopause
An Atlas of Contraception
An Atlas of Endometriosis
An Atlas of Ultrasonography in Obstetrics and Gynecology
An Atlas of Practical Radiology
An Atlas of Psoriasis
An Atlas of Lung Infections
An Atlas of Transvaginal Color Doppler
An Atlas of Child Health
An Atlas of Infective Endocarditis
An Atlas of Rheumatology
An Atlas of Epilepsy
An Atlas of HIV and AIDS-related Diseases
An Atlas of Practical Dermatology
An Atlas of Laser Operative Laparoscopy and Hysteroscopy
An Atlas of Atherosclerosis
An Atlas of Eye Diseases
An Atlas of Cutaneous Growths
An Atlas of Myocardial Infarction

Series Foreword

The art of effective diagnosis is one that relies to a considerable degree – although certainly not exclusively – on the recognition of visual signs and manifestations of disease. The objective of the Series is to provide a practical aid to diagnosis by illustrating and explaining the wide range of visual signs that a physician needs to be aware of in current medical practice.

Whilst the visual manifestations of disease themselves remain constant, the development of new techniques of invasive and non-invasive diagnosis mean that new images are frequently being added to the range of visual material that the diagnostician must be familiar with: ultrasound, radiology, magnetic resonance imaging, endoscopy and photomicrography all provide examples of this kind of material. It is the intention of this Series to document, where appropriate, the result of such techniques and to explain and elucidate their relevance – in addition to documenting all the more standard visual images.

The Series is also distinctive in that individual volumes will focus on carefully selected, specific topics, which can be covered in some detail – rather than on generalized and broadly-based subject areas that could not easily be covered so thoroughly.

The authors contributing to the Series have all been selected for their special expertise in their own chosen fields, their access to outstanding visual material and their ability to explain the significance of it in an effective and lucid way. Finally, particular emphasis is being placed on achieving a very high quality of colour reproduction in the printing process itself in order to do full justice to the wide variety of visual images presented.

It is hoped that this carefully structured and systematic approach to the visually significant aspects of medicine will make a valuable and ongoing contribution to good diagnostic practice.

Foreword

Trauma is the plague of youth, accounting for the majority of deaths in the first four decades of life, and for double this number of cases of permanent disability. In the UK it has been estimated that 24% of all individuals involved in road traffic accidents develop a disability that lasts for at least 6 months. These figures equate to a substantial loss of national revenue in this potentially productive age group, and highlight one of the most expensive problems for a National Health Service.

The deaths are trimodal in nature: immediate, early and delayed. Immediate deaths are due to organ disruption, particularly the brain, heart and lungs; the time factor denies potential medical improvement of this group. Early deaths are within a few hours and are due to visceral laceration, blood loss, and haemorrhage into the cranium, chest and abdomen. The period is often termed 'the golden hour' for the critically injured and offers the main opportunity for influencing outcomes. Late deaths occur after 3–4 days, extending to a few weeks. They are related to sepsis and organ failure; they are markedly affected by the quality of resuscitation and treatment in the early hours after trauma. Whereas the importance of accident prevention cannot be over-emphasized, multiple injuries must be managed by knowledgeable and skilled individuals if they are to minimize death and morbidity.

In recent years, there has been an explosive development in trauma training of medical, nursing and paramedical personnel. The leader in the educational field has been the Advanced Trauma Life Support (ATLS) Course adopted by the American College of Surgeons. The course was initially targeted at clinicians who do not regularly manage trauma patients, yet may be required to evaluate and manage severely injured patients, particularly during the golden hour period. Subsequent work has shown it to be applicable to all health care providers dealing with trauma. The ATLS system has set national standards for trauma programmes in the USA, facilitating training and certification. The system is now being developed in Europe, South Africa, Australia and the Middle East.

The ATLS course is a comprehensive, systematized, concise means of acute trauma management. It comprises rapid accurate assessment, immediate resuscitative measures to treat life-threatening conditions, defines management priorities and initiates a logical sequential treatment regime. It is not the only possible method of trauma management but it does provide a well-tried ordered pathway, allowing individuals to follow preset instructions. The unified approach allows for the steps to be undertaken by an individual, or a team working together, without any problems of conflicting management regimes.

This book follows the ATLS philosophy, taking a pragmatic, prescriptive and didactic approach to promote its international message. In no way does it replace the ATLS course or the essential component of practical experience in trauma management. However, it complements and reinforces these teachings. The text is concise and informative but the illustrations are extensive and provide a vivid, descriptive and educational sequence.

The book will provide a continuous reminder of the principles of trauma management, retaining the bubbling enthusiasm that ATLS courses generate in the medic. It is also ideal reading for nursing and paramedical personnel involved with the management of severe injury. It will ensure that individuals can confidently implement basic trauma skills, and that the team is always prepared and ready to undertake immediate trauma management. This in turn will help to reduce the current appalling degree of unnecessary death and disability generated in young trauma victims.

Professor of Vascular Surgery   *John S. P. Lumley*
St. Bartholomew's Hospital
London, UK
and
Immediate Past President
International College of Surgeons

Preface

Trauma is the modern epidemic and its management may take several forms. The objective of this book is to provide an illustrated guide which marries together the theory and practice of trauma management. This text acknowledges the internationally recognized 'Advanced Trauma Life Support' system promulgated by the American College of Surgeons. We are indebted to the American College of Surgeons for the privilege of using their system as the architecture of this Atlas.

We should like to acknowledge the inspiration, help and advice of the following individuals in the production of this book: Professor Peter Cull, Department of Informatics and Clinical Skills, St. Bartholomew's Hospital, Professor John Landon, Department of Chemical Pathology, St. Bartholomew's Hospital, Professor John Lumley, Department of Surgery, St. Bartholomew's Hospital, Mr Carlos Perez-Avila OBE., Consultant, Accident and Emergency Department, The Royal Sussex County Hospital, Brighton and Mr Robin Touquet, Consultant, Accident and Emergency, St. Mary's Hospital, London.

Bridget A. Landon
Peter Driscoll
John D. Goodall

Introduction: the management of a trauma patient

There are three stages in the management of a trauma victim based upon the ATLS (Advanced Trauma Life Support) system of care:

Primary survey and resuscitation
Secondary survey
Definitive care

The objectives of the first of these stages are to hunt out *and* treat any immediately life-threatening condition. This follows the ABC format:

Airway and cervical spine control
Breathing
Circulation
Dysfunction
Exposure

When a trauma team is available, several of these tasks can be carried out simultaneously. However, the list order should be followed if the clinician is working alone.

The objectives of the Secondary survey are to identify all the potentially life-threatening conditions and assess all the other injuries so that an appropriate management plan can be developed. This is then put into effect during the Definitive care phase.

1
Prehospital care and the mechanism of injury

Usually the patient at the incident site is initially managed by ambulance and paramedical personnel. However, an emergency medical and nursing squad can be of benefit in complicated cases, particularly when there are problems of entrapment. It is essential that all these people are adequately trained to work safely and effectively in this potentially hostile environment.

Prehospital care has the same objectives as that found in the resuscitation room. However, the rescuer must not put himself or his colleagues at risk. Therefore, only when the scene has been made safe (or the patient transferred to a safe area) can the assessment and resuscitation commence. This entails clearing and securing the airway whilst maintaining in-line cervical stabilization (Figure 1). Following this, adequate ventilation, haemorrhage control and early insertion of intravenous lines can be carried out (Figure 2). The posture of the patient and overt blood loss at the scene must be noted. It is also essential that the initial vital signs are recorded (respiratory rate, heart rate, blood pressure, Glasgow Coma Score) and reassessed frequently. Consequently, any change in the patient's state can be noted.

In addition to these A, B and Cs, it is important to consider the pain, anxiety and distress which the patient will be experiencing. Appropriate analgesics, splintage and a supportive attitude may be required.

Clumsy extrication and transfer from the site of the incident can jeopardize the spinal cord, exacerbate blood loss and increase soft tissue damage around fractures. These secondary injuries can be prevented by stabilizing the patient before transfer and utilizing the skills of the emergency services. To this end, scoop stretchers, short (Figure 3) and long (Figure 4) spinal boards, splints and pneumatic antishock garments (Figure 5) may be used.

It is very important that prehospital personnel record details of the incident and the environment in which it occurred (Figure 6). This is crucial for the future management of the patient in the Accident and Emergency department. Potential patterns of injuries are suggested once the mechanism of the injury is known.

PATTERNS OF INJURY
Blunt injury
Blunt injury can occur in a variety of circumstances, for example, road traffic accidents, industrial accidents and falls. Such injuries involve impact forces in which the body tissues are subjected to deformation. Pressure changes can rupture hollow viscera and shatter solid organs. Damage is most pronounced where structures are only anchored at one place, for example, the main bronchi (one inch from the carina) and the aortic arch (level of the ligamentum arteriosum).

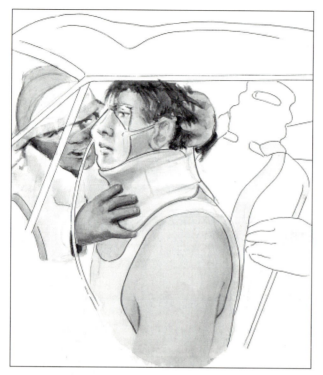

Figure 1 Cervical spine immobilization

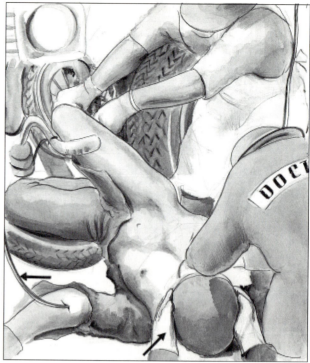

Figure 2 In-line immobilization of cervical spine and setting up of intravenous lines

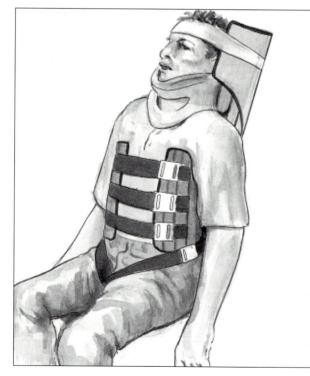

Figure 3 The short spinal board

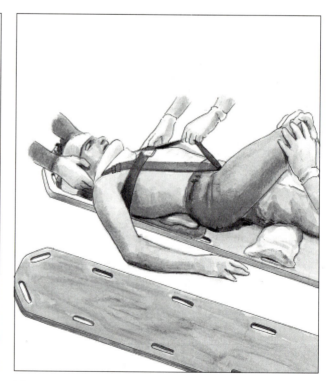

Figure 4 The long spinal board

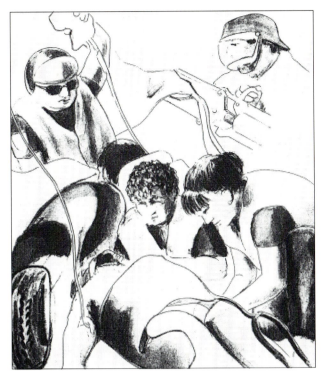

Figure 5 Pneumatic antishock garments

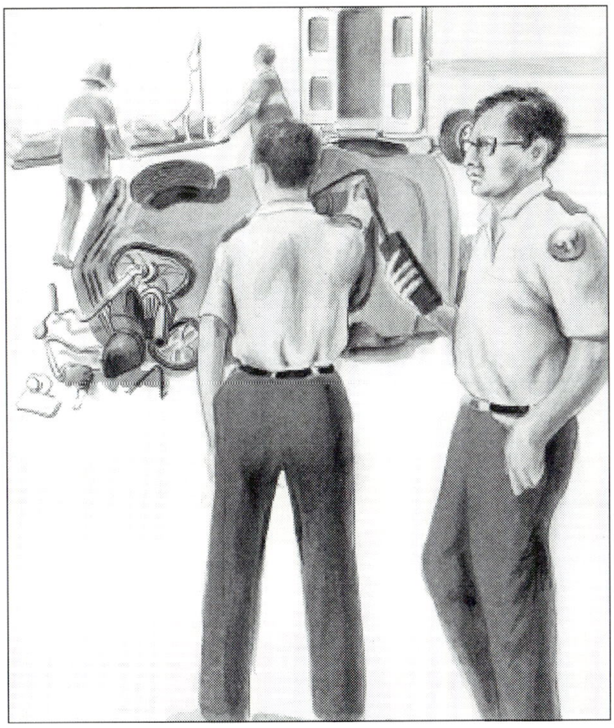

Figure 6 Prehospital personnel should record details of the incident and environment

Depending on the degree and direction of the force, bone can fracture, allowing energy to dissipate into the local soft tissue and cause further damage.

Motor car accidents usually involve either head-on collisions or an oblique blow producing rotational forces. Pure lateral and rear-shunting impacts are less frequent. Vehicle deformation and fatalities at the scene are indicators of the force of impact. Head-on collisions can produce a spectrum of injuries when the occupant strikes the steering column, dashboard, windscreen and footwell (Figure 7). These include thoracic and abdominal damage, injuries of the trachea, fractures of the knees and femurs and dislocation of the hips. In the absence of a seat belt, severe facial fractures, lacerations and head injuries can occur. If a patient is thrown from a vehicle, his chance of a significant injury is increased by 300%.

Rotational forces from glancing impacts dissipate the energy through turning as well as linear motion.

These are better tolerated but the injuries are similar to those found in a frontal collision.

When the weaker lateral wall of a vehicle is hit, intrusion commonly occurs (Figure 8). This can produce significant skull, cervical spine, thoracic, abdominal, pelvic and upper limb injuries on the appropriate side.

Rear-end collisions are a potent cause of cervical injury. Hyperextension against a low head rest, followed by hyperflexion, is a well-recognized mechanism (Figure 9).

Multiple complex forces are imparted when a car rolls over (Figure 10). These can be compounded by intrusion of the vehicle roof, leading to crushing of the head, trunk and limbs. These are more likely to occur if the patient was not wearing a seat belt or if the vehicle was a convertible.

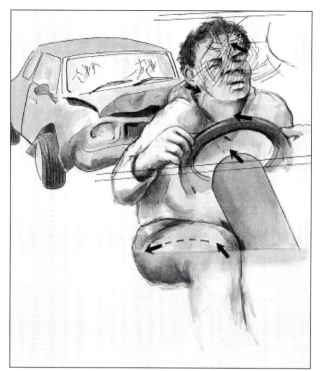

Figure 7 Head-on collision in a motor car accident

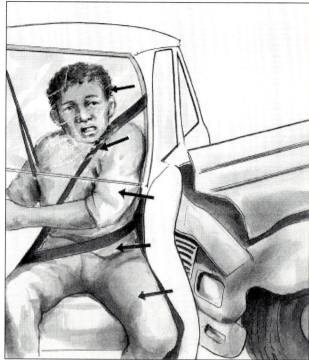

Figure 8 Lateral impact in a motor car accident

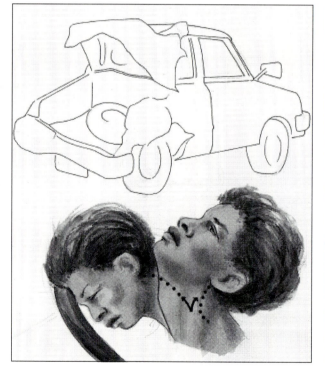

Figure 9 Rear end collision in a motor car accident

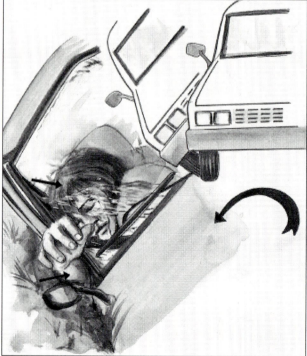

Figure 10 The rollover pattern of injury consisting of trapped limbs and head injury

Motorcycle accidents are well known to be associated with severe multiple injuries. Simple collisions with the side of the bike can cause crushing injuries to the lower limbs (Figure 11). The rider(s) become vulnerable to striking any stationary object at the roadside once they become dislodged. When thrown forwards, the handlebars may produce femoral or pelvic fractures (Figure 12). Thoracic and particularly brachial plexus damage occurs as the trunk and apex of the shoulder strike the road (Figure 13). The laceration to the skin from abrasive forces is reduced considerably by leather protective clothing. Well maintained, modern motorcycle helmets are also of great value.

Pedestrians involved in road traffic accidents can sustain severe, life-threatening injuries. The common, side-on impact produces characteristic bumper fractures of the tibia and disruption of the knee ligaments. As the torso is projected over the bonnet, the pelvis, spine, chest and head may also be injured (Figures 14 and 15).

The pattern of injuries associated with a fall from a height depends on the objects struck en route and the mode of landing (Figure 16). In the 'feet first' approach, fractures of the os calcis, lower tibia, pelvis, spine and base of skull may occur. In addition, there can be rupture of the main bronchi and dissection of the thoracic aorta. It is also important to consider why the person fell – was the building on fire or was it a suicide attempt? In such cases, associated burns or a drug overdose should be considered.

Penetrating trauma

The severity of this type of injury is dependent on the site and amount of tissue damaged. The latter is dependent on how much energy is imparted to the tissues by the missile. High-energy transfers lead to cavitation, marked tissue destruction and contamination. Tumbling of the bullet and ricocheting off bony structures allow further energy loss and consequently more damage.

It is important to remember that knife wounds can be fatal if they are in a vital area. Furthermore, the size of the wound gives no clue to its actual depth.

Blast injuries

Following the detonation of an explosive, a pressure (shock) wave moves rapidly from the epicentre causing physical disruption to any surface it hits. With certain types of explosives, this can be associated with intense heat. The shock wave is quickly followed by a blast wind which carries thousands of sharp projectiles from the bomb itself as well as from surrounding structures (e.g. furniture). Consequently, bomb blasts can produce a combination of blunt, penetrating and burn injuries.

Burns

Burns can result from the flash of a combustion, a secondary ignition of clothing or chemical contamination. Removal of clothing and specific measures should be considered early (Figure 17). Inhalation of smoke is a common and serious accompaniment (Figure 18).

Near-drowning incidents

Incidents of near-drowning may be associated with cervical spine injury and hypothermia.

TRANSPORT

Transport is usually carried out by land ambulances. However, the helicopter should be considered when the scene is inaccessible to the ordinary ambulance or when a long transfer time is anticipated.

Whichever method is used, the A, B and Cs must be completed and the patient monitored continuously throughout his journey.

A warning should be given to the receiving hospital as to the patient's age, sex, injuries, vital signs, treatment and response. An estimated time of arrival is also important.

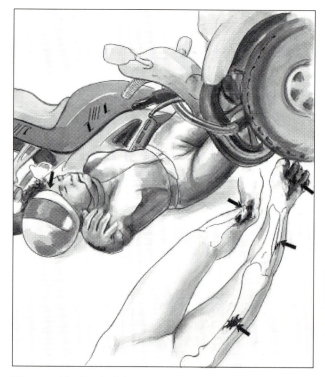

Figure 11 Crush injury to lower limb in a motorcycle accident

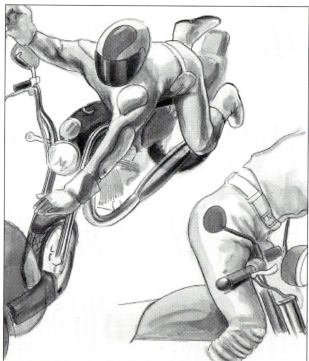

Figure 12 Handlebar injury to abdomen, pelvis and femurs

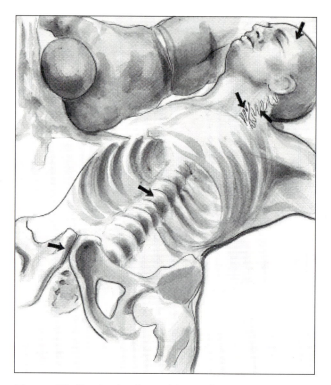

Figure 13 Ejection leading to injury to head, brachial plexus, spine and pelvis

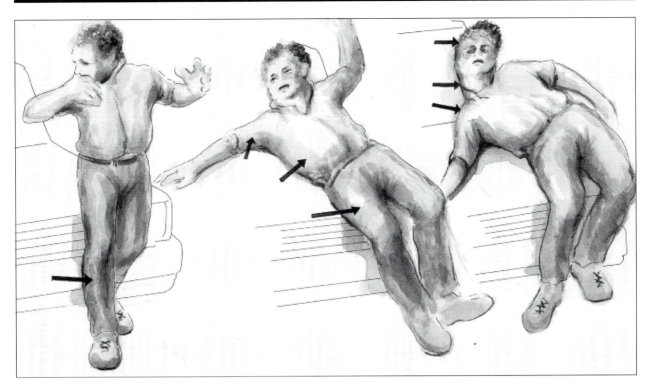

Figure 14 Pattern of injury to an adult pedestrian in a motor car accident caused by an oblique blow

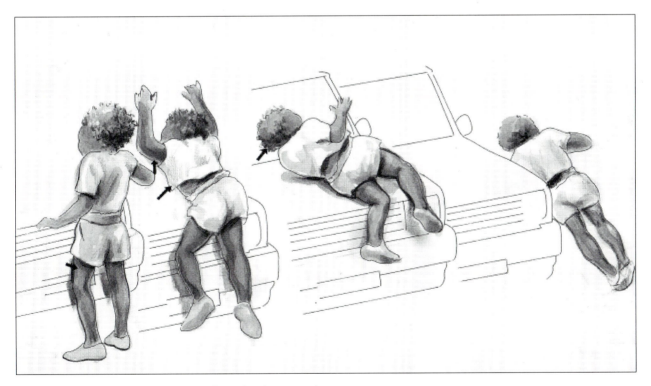

Figure 15 Pattern of injury to a juvenile pedestrian caused by a head-on collision

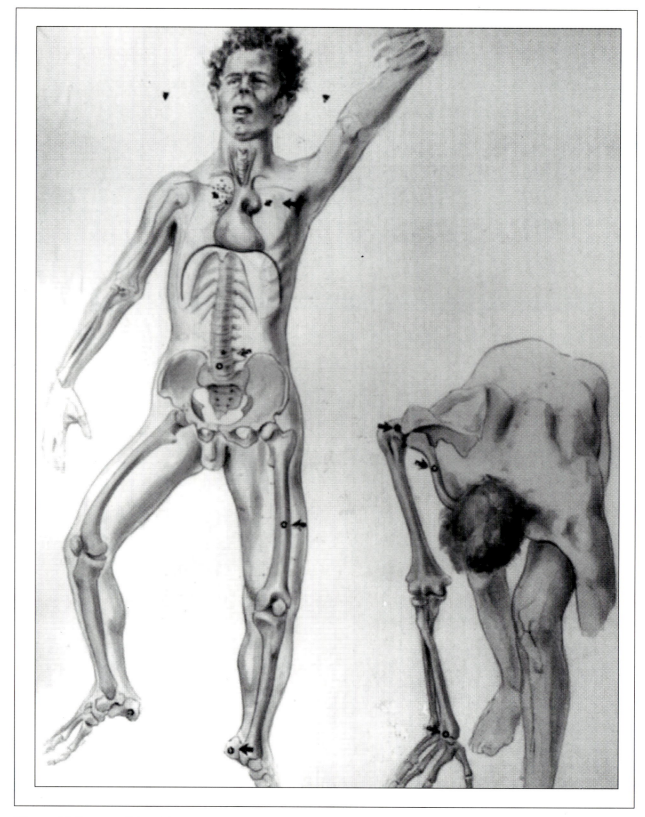

Figure 16 Pattern of blunt injury caused by a fall

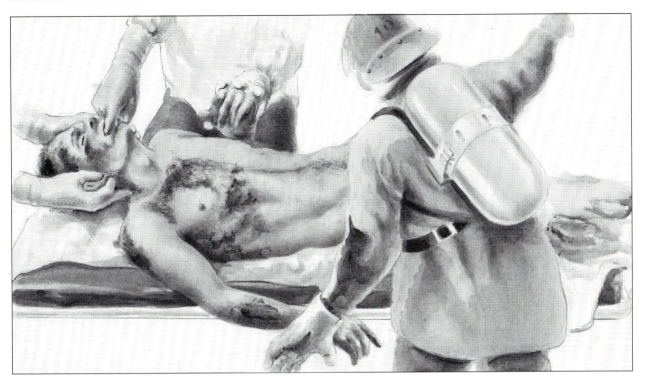

Figure 17 Early removal of clothing for burn injury

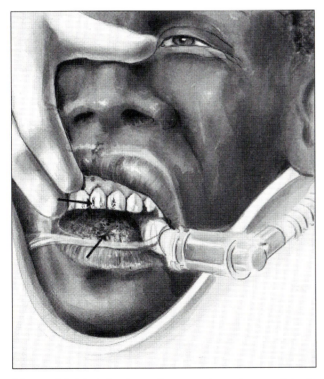

Figure 18 Inhalation burn: there may be carbon particles in the mouth and on the teeth

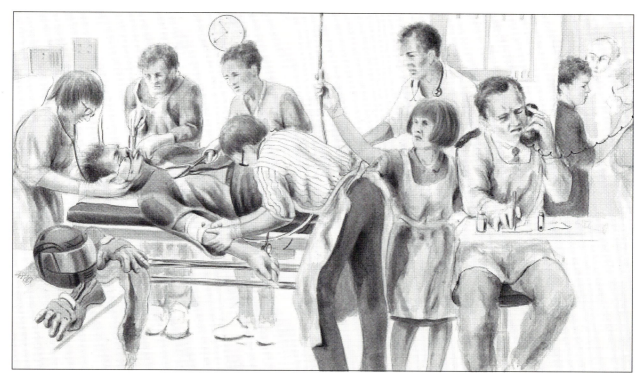

Figure 19 The trauma team

TRAUMA TEAM

With pre-warning, a team of medical and nursing personnel can be assembled (Figure 19). The optimum number is between five and ten. However, it is essential that each member knows what tasks he/she has to perform. One of the team leader's functions is to ensure that the tasks are carried out simultaneously and effectively once the patient arrives. The team consists of a leader, an experienced doctor; a nurse leader; an anaesthetist and a nurse for airway management; a doctor and two nurses for circulation management; and a nurse to care for the relatives.

2

Airway and cervical spine control

The most important aspect in the management of the trauma patient is ensuring that the airway is clear and secure (Figure 1). However, during these activities the potentially unstable cervical spine must not be moved.

BASIC AIRWAY MANAGEMENT AND CERVICAL SPINE CONTROL

Simultaneous assessment of the airway, with stabilization of the cervical spine, is best achieved by holding the patient's head with both hands and asking, 'Are you alright?' (Figure 2).

The head can also be stabilized from below by an assistant (Figure 3). This arrangement is used when motorcycle helmets are removed (see before). It also gives the clinician better access to the patient's airway.

A sensible reply with a normal voice indicates that the airway is patent and the patient's brain is being adequately perfused. This type of trauma victim can maintain his own airway. However, he still requires an oxygen mask and reservoir, with a flow rate of 15 l/min (Figure 4). The neck can then be definitively stabilized (see later).

No attempt at a reply usually indicates that the patient is unconscious. A rapid assessment of the ventilation should then be carried out by the 'look, listen and feel' technique (Figure 5). If this is found to be inadequate, artificial ventilation must be commenced once the airway has been cleared and secured.

An impaired response could indicate that there is an obstruction of the airway. The resulting hypoxia can lead to tachypnoea, the use of the accessory muscles of ventilation, agitation, confusion and stridor.

It should be remembered that patients will try to sit up if their airway is unstable and obstructs when they lie down (Figure 6).

The commonest cause of airway obstruction is due to the tongue sliding backwards (Figure 7) and occluding the pharynx. Other causes consist of fractures of the mandible (Figure 8) or maxilla, vomit, a torrential haemorrhage in the mouth or a foreign body occluding the larynx.

In most cases, the tongue can be pulled forward, and a patent airway created, by using the chin lift or jaw thrust techniques. The cervical spine is not moved in either of these manoeuvres if they are carried out correctly. In the chin lift procedure, the index and middle fingers pull the mandible forward as the thumb assists and pushes down the lower lip and jaw (Figure 9). The jaw thrust technique is carried out by placing

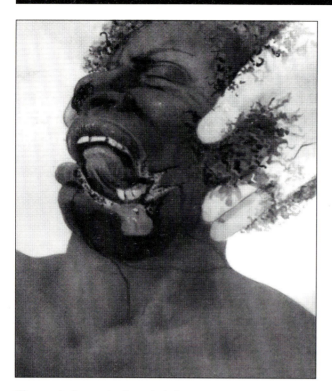

Figure 1 A grossly disrupted airway

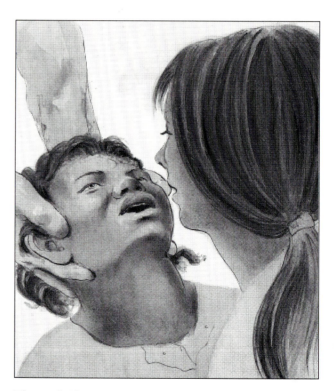

Figure 2 'Are you alright?'

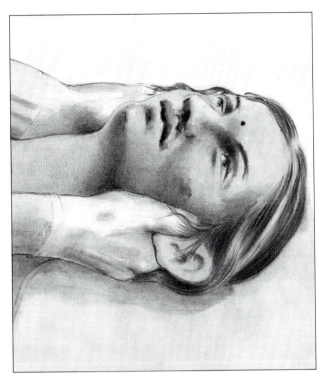

Figure 3 The head stabilized from below

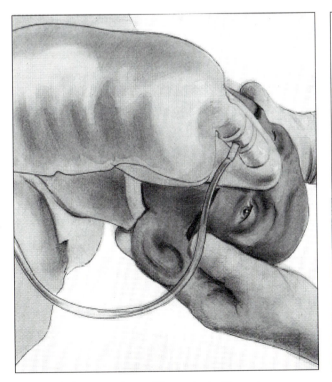

Figure 4 A patent airway. The patient still needs an oxygen mask and reservoir

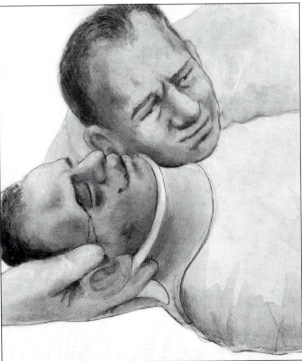

Figure 5 The 'look, listen and feel' technique

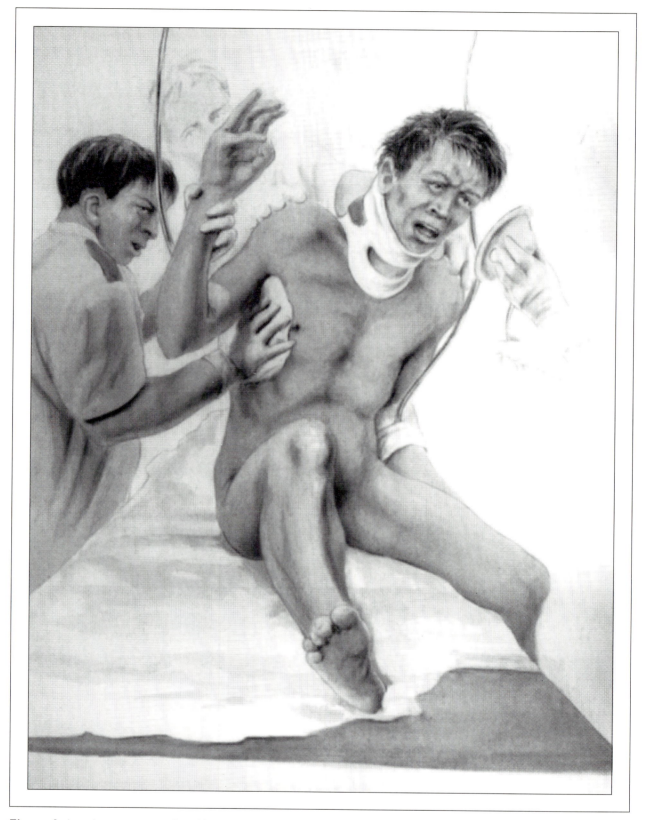

Figure 6 A patient may try to sit up if his airway is unstable and is obstructed when he lies down

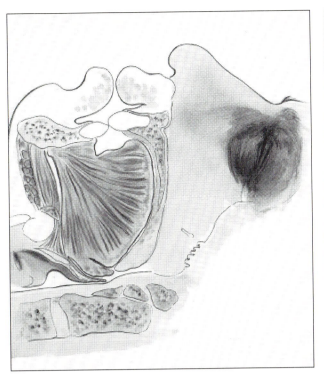

Figure 7 The tongue is occluding the pharynx and the epiglottis is occluding the larynx

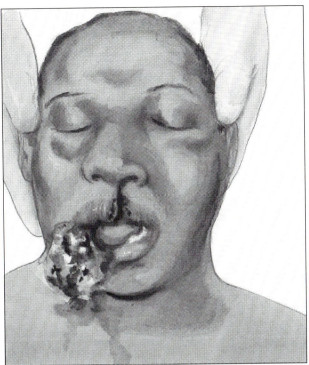

Figure 8 Airway obstruction due to fractured mandible

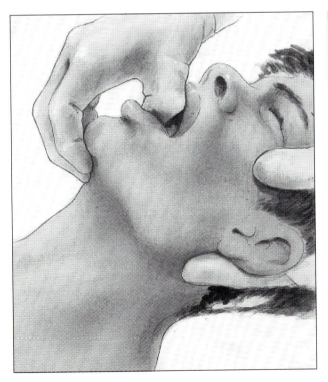

Figure 9 The chin lift procedure

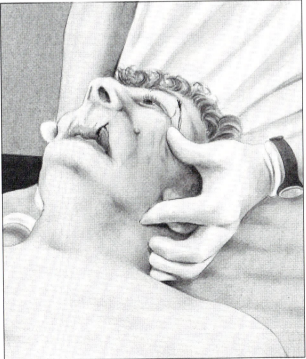

Figure 10 The jaw thrust technique

both hands behind the angles of the patient's jaw with the thumbs placed over the malar prominences. As the thumbs push down, the fingers lift the mandible forward (Figure 10).

Ventilation should then be reassessed using the 'look, listen and feel' technique (Figure 11). If these techniques fail to clear the airway, the mouth must be opened and inspected for loose or lost teeth, foreign bodies or vomitus (Figure 12). Any vomitus should be removed with a rigid sucker (Yankauer) (Figure 13). Solid material is more easily removed with a pair of Magill forceps.

Examination of the mouth will reveal if the cough and gag reflexes are present. A nasopharyngeal airway will be better tolerated if the pharyngeal reflexes are still present. A well lubricated tube, having an internal diameter of 6–8 mm, is inserted into a patent nostril (Figure 14). It is pushed backwards, parallel to the hard palate, with a slight rotary action. A safety pin is then inserted through the end of the tube to prevent it being inhaled.

If the pharyngeal reflexes are absent, an oropharyngeal airway (Guedel) should be inserted to help keep the tongue from sliding backward. The guide to the correct size is given by the distance from the corner of the jaw to the middle of the teeth (Figure 15). The Guedel airway is inserted upside down until the tip reaches the hard palate. It is then rotated through 180° and fully inserted until the flange lies in front of the teeth (Figure 16). Jaw thrust or chin lift can then be recommenced and the adequacy of ventilation reassessed by the 'look, listen and feel' method (Figure 17).

BASIC MANAGEMENT OF BREATHING

If the patient is breathing spontaneously, a close-fitting mask with reservoir should be placed over the

patient's face and connected to an oxygen flow of 15 l/min (Figure 18). A self-inflating bag, connected to a non-rebreathing valve, mask and reservoir bag, is required in cases of apnoea or inadequate ventilation. An oxygen flow of 15 l/min should be attached to the reservoir bag (Figure 19). The facemask is held in place with the thumb and index finger, whilst the other three fingers perform a jaw thrust and chin lift manoeuvre (Figure 20). The patient should be ventilated at 12–15 breaths/min.

ADVANCED AIRWAY CONTROL

Basic control of the airway may prove to be inadequate or impossible in five trauma situations:

(1) Loss of protective reflexes;

(2) Disrupted airway, e.g. severe facial trauma;

(3) Specific need for ventilation, e.g. head injury;

(4) Compromise of normal respiratory mechanism;

(5) Anticipated future airway obstruction.

Before intubating the patient, it is important that all the necessary equipment is laid out appropriately and checked (Figure 21). The patient should be preoxygenated and the cervical spine stabilized by an assistant throughout the procedure. To prevent migration down the trachea and bronchi, loose teeth should be removed prior to the intubation procedure. The patient should not be deprived of oxygen for greater than 30 s. If intubation has not been achieved, the patient must be re-oxygenated before a further attempt is made.

Oral intubation

This technique is recommended in those patients who are apnoeic and have no cervical spine injury. The clinician must have the skill to carry out this technique. The laryngoscope is lifted in the left hand and the patient's mouth opened with a scissor action of the

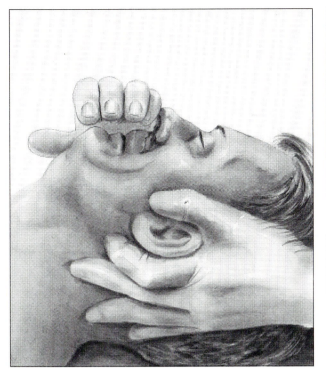

Figure 11 Reassessment of ventilation

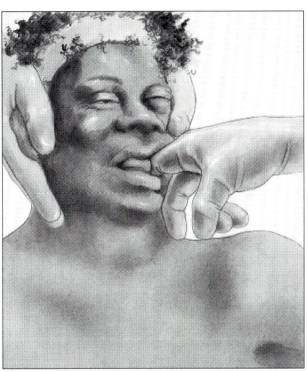

Figure 12 Mouth inspection

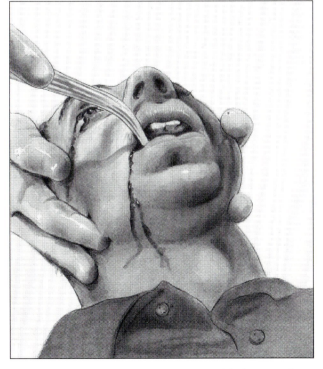

Figure 13 Removal of vomitus with the Yankauer sucker

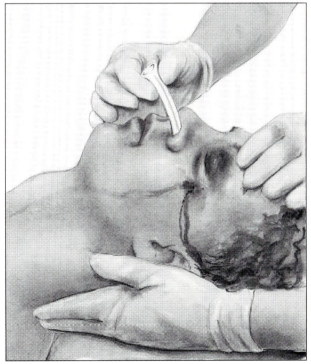

Figure 14 Insertion of a nasopharyngeal airway

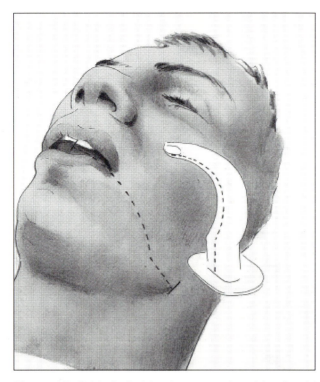

Figure 15 Guide for judging the correct size of the Guedal airway

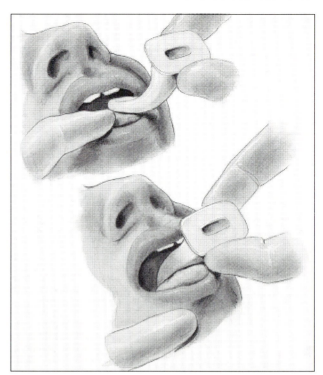

Figure 16 Insertion of the Guedal airway

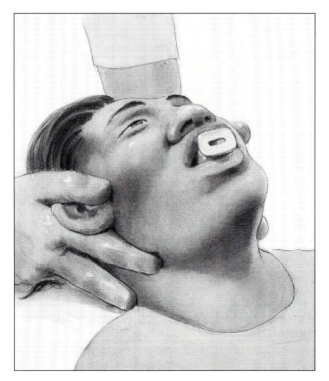

Figure 17 Recommencement of chin lift or jaw thrust and reassessment of ventilation

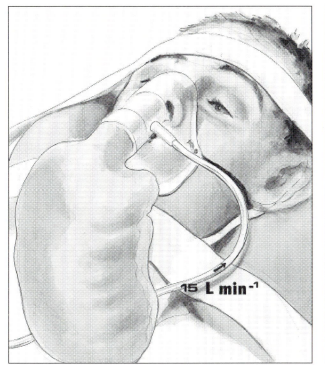

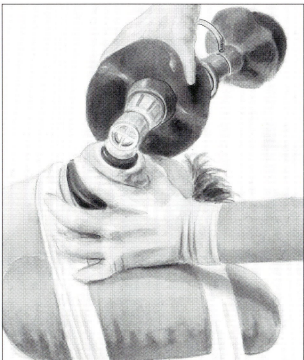

Figure 18 A close fitting oxygen mask with reservoir is placed over the patient's face

Figure 19 In case of apnoea or inadequate ventilation, a self-inflating bag is required

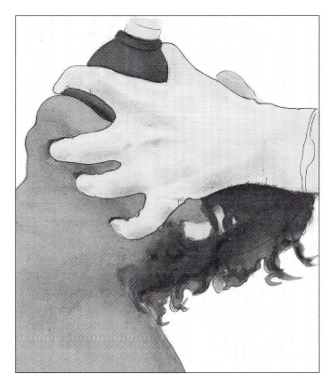

Figure 20 Correct placement of a face mask

right thumb and index finger (Figure 22). The blade is advanced down the right side of the tongue until the tip comes to lie in the vallecula. The tongue is displaced to the left (Figure 23). Force is then applied in the direction of the handle of the laryngoscope. There should be no wrist action as this can cause the upper teeth to be damaged by the proximal part of the blade (Figure 24). This action brings the vocal cords and laryngeal inlet into view (Figure 25). The tracheal tube can then be inserted. Only the posterior aspects of the vocal cords are usually visible because cervical spine control is being maintained. If this prohibits intubation, a gum-elastic bougie should initially be inserted through the vocal cords (Figure 26). The tracheal tube can then be slid over the bougie (Figure 27).

Once in place, the tube cuff can be inflated and the patient ventilated. The chest should be assessed for symmetry of air entry, absence of gastric air entry and the measurement of the end-tidal carbon dioxide (Figure 28). If there is doubt about the correct placement of the tube, the cuff must be deflated and the tube withdrawn. The patient must then be pre-oxygenated again before placement is re-attempted.

Nasal intubation

This technique is recommended if the patient is breathing spontaneously and there is a possibility of a cervical spine injury. The clinician must have the skill to carry out this technique.

The procedure is carried out whilst maintaining in-line cervical stabilization. The nasal passages are sprayed with a local anaesthetic containing a vasoconstrictor agent (Figure 29).

The nasal endotracheal tube is lubricated and inserted into a patent nostril in a similar manner to the insertion of the nasopharyngeal airway (Figure 30). When the tip of the tube is in the pharynx, the clinician should listen for the expiratory noise (Figure 31). The tube is pushed in the direction of maximum noise, as

this will position the tip just above the larynx. At the moment of inspiration, the tube is advanced into the trachea. If unsuccessful, the thyroid cartilage can be pressed backwards and directed upwards (Figure 32). The correct placement of the tube is then assessed by the methods described previously. It can then be secured and the patient ventilated at 12–15 breaths/min with 100% oxygen flowing at 15 l/min.

Cricoid pressure

The aim of this technique is to minimize the chance of regurgitation and aspiration of stomach contents during intubation or when the patient is being artificially ventilated. Direct, midline pressure is placed on the cricoid ring by an assistant (Figure 33).

Cricoid pressure compresses the oesophagus between the 6th cervical vertebra and the cricoid ring (Figure 34). Cricoid pressure should not be removed until the tube is in the trachea and the cuff inflated. The exception to this rule is when the patient *actively* vomits. In this situation, the pressure must be released as there is a risk of oesophageal rupture. The patient is then tipped head down and the mouth sucked out whilst cervical stabilization is maintained (Figure 35). The patient can be turned onto his side only if a spinal injury has been excluded.

SURGICAL AIRWAY

Occasionally, endotracheal intubation is not possible because of oedema or trauma producing a complete airway obstruction (Figure 36).

Needle cricothyroidotomy

This type of patient can be temporarily ventilated, using a needle cricothyroidotomy.

The equipment must be checked prior to carrying out this procedure (Figure 37). It is important that the

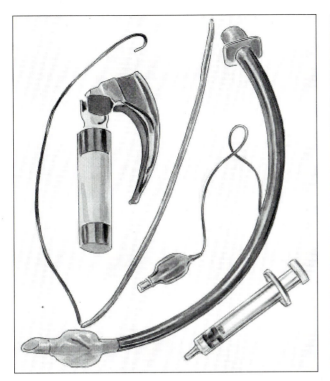

Figure 21 Equipment required for intubation

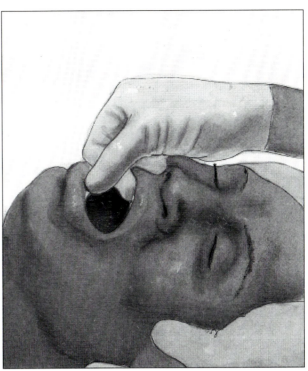

Figure 22 The scissor action in oral intubation

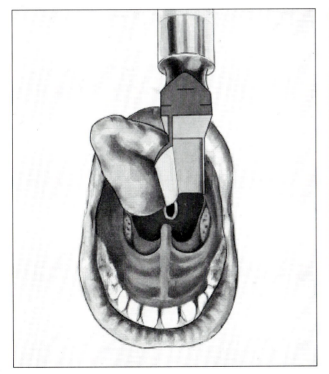

Figure 23 Insertion of the blade of the laryngoscope

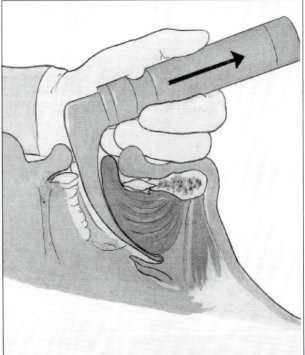

Figure 24 Force is applied in the direction of the handle

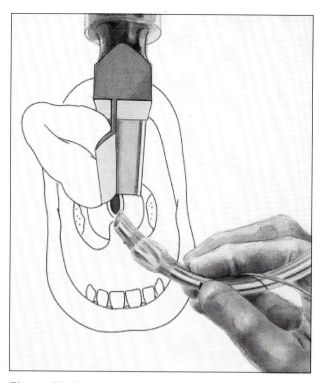

Figure 25 The vocal cords and laryngeal inlet are brought into view

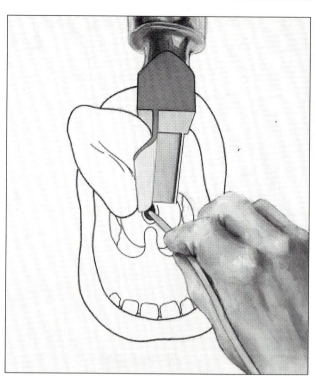

Figure 26 Insertion of a gum-elastic bougie

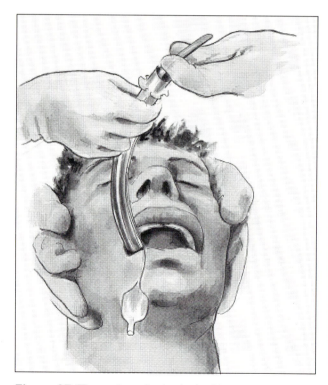

Figure 27 The endotracheal tube is slid over the bougie

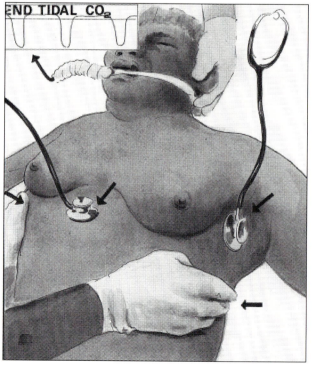

Figure 28 After ventilation, the chest is assessed for symmetry of movement, the end-tidal carbon dioxide is monitored and the axillae and epigastrum are auscultated

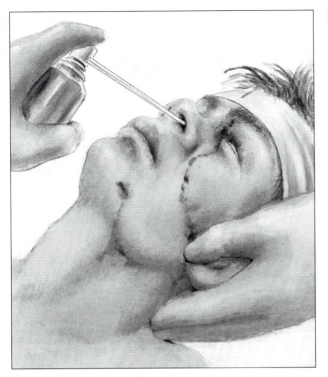

Figure 29 The nasal passages are sprayed with local anaesthetic

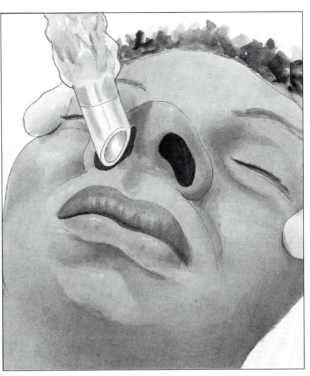

Figure 30 Insertion of the nasal endotracheal tube into the nostril

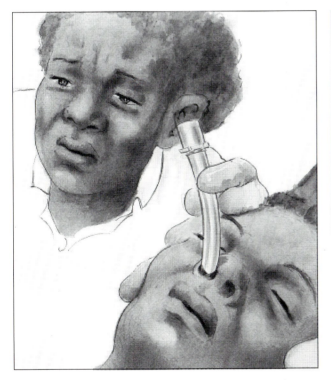

Figure 31 The clinician listens for the expiratory noise

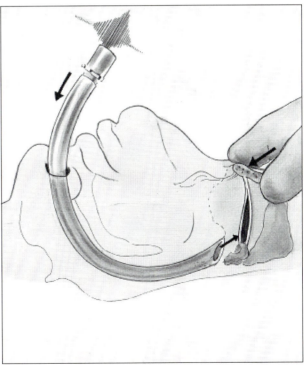

Figure 32 Advancement of tube into the trachea

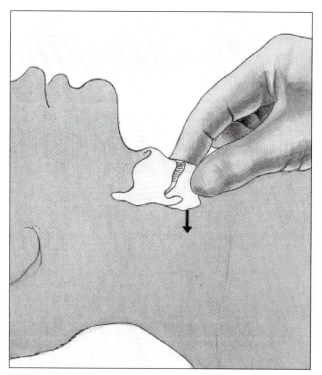

Figure 33 Application of cricoid pressure

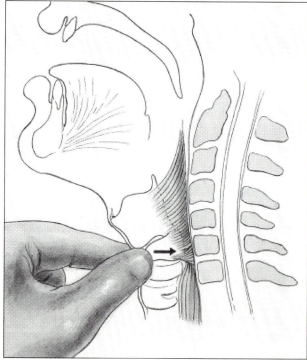

Figure 34 Compression of oesophagus between the 6th cervical vertebra and the cricoid ring

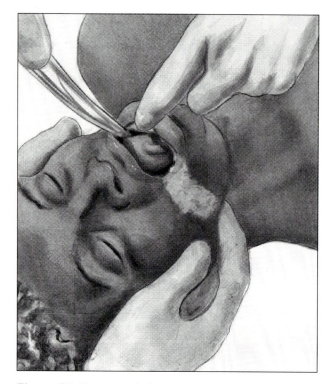

Figure 35 Remove cricoid pressure and use suction if the patient vomits

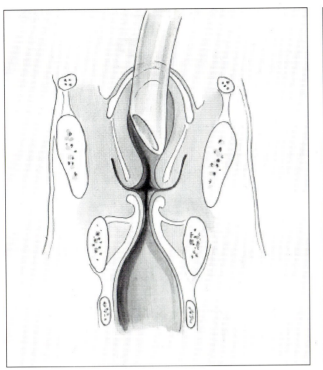

Figure 36 Obstruction of the larynx by oedema

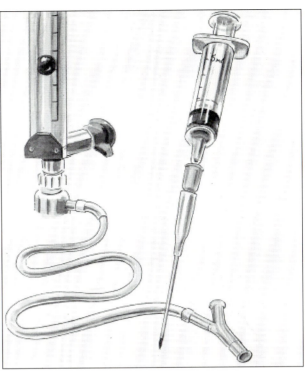

Figure 37 Equipment for needle cricothyroidotomy, consisting of a 5 ml syringe, 12-gauge cannula, oxygen tubing with a 'Y' connector and a rotameter

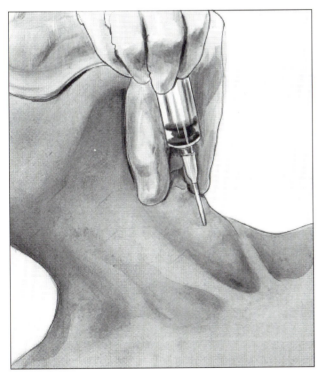

Figure 38 Insertion of cannula with aspiration of air

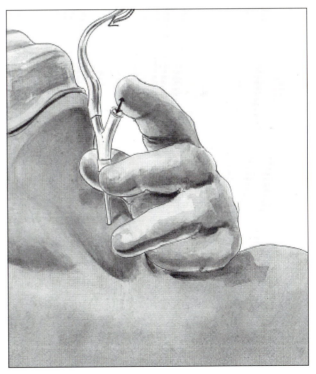

Figure 39 Occlusion of the free limb of the 'Y' connector

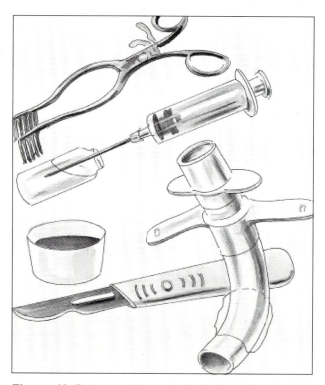

Figure 40 Equipment for surgical cricothyroidotomy, consisting of skin prep, local anaesthetic with adrenaline, scalpel, self-retainer and tracheostomy tube

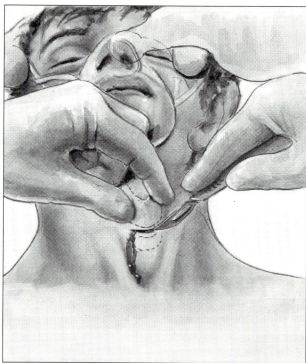

Figure 41 The incision into the cricothyroid membrane

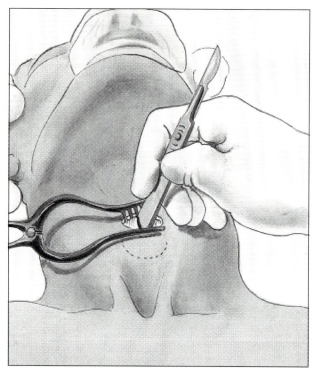

Figure 42 The creation of a track

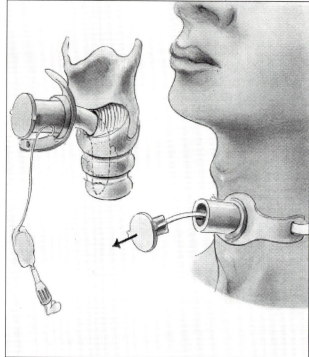

Figure 43 Insertion of the tracheostomy tube

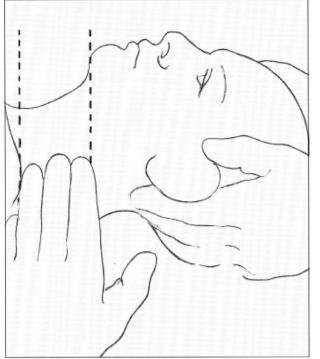

Figure 44 Correct sizing of cervical collar

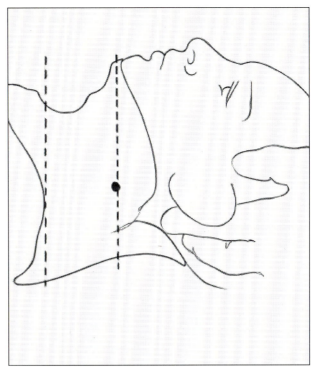

Figure 45 Positioning of cervical collar

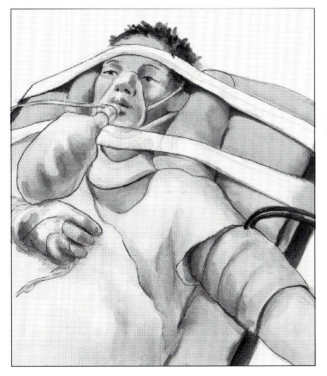

Figure 46 Prevention of rotational movements of head, using sandbags and tape, when an oxygen mask is required

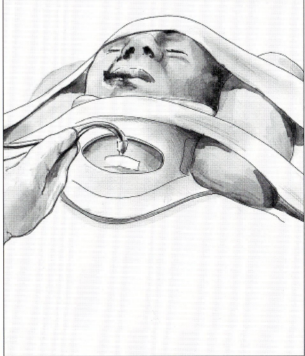

Figure 47 Prevention of rotational movement of head when a tracheostomy tube is in position

patient continues to receive a high flow of oxygen during the insertion of the needle.

A 12- or 14-gauge intravenous cannula is inserted through the cricothyroid membrane in a caudal direction (Figure 38). Air is aspirated to make sure the cannula is in the trachea. Due to the obstruction, the larynx moves in a cephalo-caudal manner. The thyroid cartilage must therefore be stabilized during this procedure. The needle is withdrawn and connected to oxygen tubing with a 'Y' connector. Oxygen, flowing at 15 l/min and at a pressure of 345 kPa, is connected. The free limb of the 'Y' connector is occluded for 1 second in 5 (Figure 39).

This technique allows the chest adequate time (4 s) to deflate. However, it fails to clear carbon dioxide effectively and so the duration of its use is 30–45 min.

Surgical cricothyroidotomy

This procedure is contraindicated if the patient is less than 12 years old, if there is evidence of laryngeal trauma or if there is an expanding cervical haematoma.

The equipment and connections must be checked before this procedure is commenced. The operator will require skin prep, local anaesthetic with adrenaline, a scalpel, a self-retainer, a syringe, tape and a tracheostomy tube (4 mm for female and 5 mm for male) (Figure 40).

The skin is cleaned and infiltrated with local anaesthetic. The thyroid cartilage is then held by the clinician and an incision made down to the cricothyroid membrane (Figure 41). A finger is then inserted into the wound to determine the exact position of the membrane. Once found, it is incised and a track is created with the scalpel and the self-retaining retractor (Figure 42). The tracheostomy tube can then be inserted by an assistant. It is vitally important to make sure the tube goes into the tracheal lumen and does not simply slide down its anterior surface (Figure 43). Once in place,

the central trocar is removed and the tube connected to a ventilatory circuit. The balloon is then inflated with air and the tube secured with the tape. Tracheal suction can be carried out with a flexible catheter.

A chest X-ray and arterial blood gas sample should be taken as soon as possible after intubation or the creation of a surgical airway.

Irrespective of which technique is required, once the airway has been cleared and secured, the cervical spine can be definitively stabilized using a semi-rigid collar of the correct size (Figure 44). This prevents flexion and extension of the neck by applying support under the chin, bracing it from the extended chest extension (Figure 45). A similar buttress functions at the occiput.

Sand bags (or litre bags of fluid) and tape are then added. The latter traverses the forehead and chin, from the sides of the trolley (Figures 46 and 47). In this way, the rotational movements of the cervical spine are eliminated.

3
Breathing and ventilation

There are six immediately life-threatening thoracic conditions which must be detected and treated during the primary survey and resuscitation phase:

(1) Airway obstruction (Figure 1);

(2) Tension pneumothorax (Figure 2);

(3) Cardiac tamponade (Figure 3);

(4) Open chest wound (Figure 4);

(5) Massive haemothorax (Figure 5);

(6) Flail chest (Figure 6).

The whole of the patient's chest has to be fully exposed so that it can be assessed by the clinician (Figure 7). The posterior aspect of the thorax is examined during the primary survey if the origin of any respiratory problem is unclear. Otherwise inspection of the back can await the secondary survey.

The thoracic wall is inspected for marks, bruising, penetrating wounds, abnormal chest movement, intercostal indrawing and respiratory rate and depth. Marks left by acceleration and deceleration forces can overlie extensive injuries. For example, the diagonal bruising pattern left by a seat belt may overlie a fractured clavicle, a thoracic aortic tear, pulmonary contusion or a pancreatic laceration (Figure 8). The steering wheel bruise over the centre of the anterior chest and epigastrium could indicate the presence of a sternal fracture, bilateral flail chest and cardiac contusion, as well as trauma to the liver, spleen, diaphragm and pancreas (Figure 9).

Well-intentioned attempts at early removal of a foreign body penetrating the chest should be resisted, as respiratory and circulatory collapse can follow.

Auscultation and percussion are used to detect any differences between the two sides of the chest. This is usually most marked over the periphery. Consequently, both axillae and the anterior chest walls are auscultated to determine if the air entry to both sides of the chest is equal (Figure 10). If the air entry is not equal, the chest is percussed to determine if one side is hyper-resonant (pneumothorax) or dull (haemothorax or a ruptured diaphragm) (Figure 11).

A good quality chest radiograph, a 12-lead ECG and an arterial blood gas analysis should be obtained as soon as possible in all trauma patients – especially if a thoracic injury is suspected.

AIRWAY OBSTRUCTION

Intercostal indrawing indicates that there is obstruction of the airway (Figure 12). The airway must be rechecked, cleared and secured using the techniques described in the previous chapter.

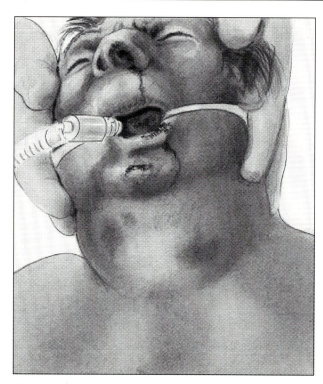

Figure 1 Airway obstruction

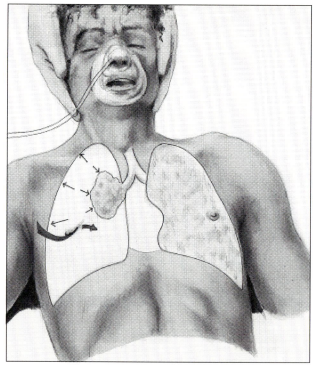

Figure 2 Tension pneumothorax

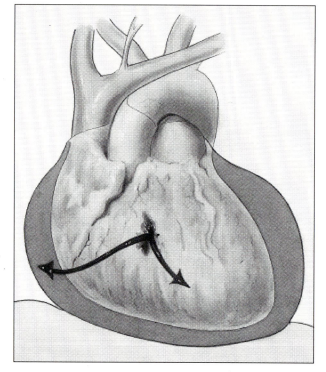

Figure 3 Cardiac tamponade

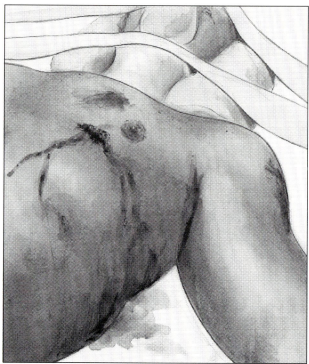

Figure 4 Open chest wound

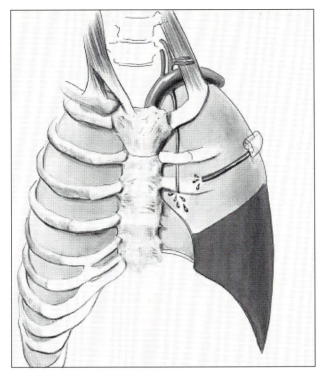

Figure 5 Massive haemothorax

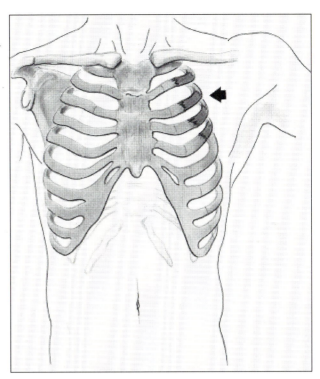

Figure 6 Flail chest

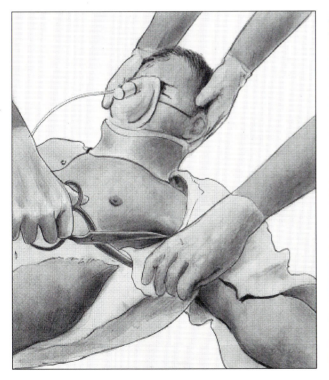

Figure 7 The chest clothes must be removed

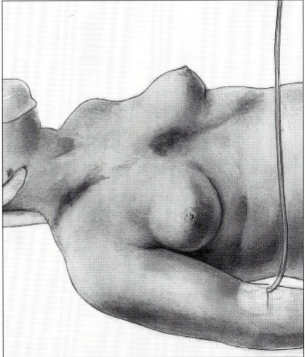

Figure 8 The diagonal bruising pattern left by a seat belt

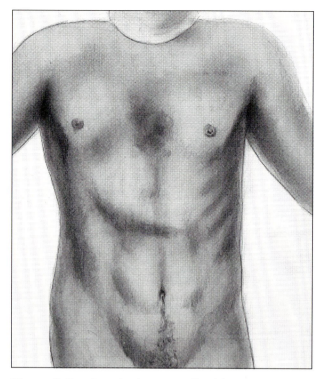

Figure 9 Steering wheel pattern of bruising

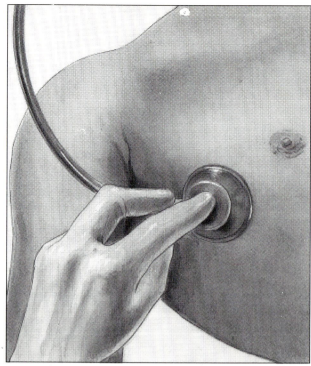

Figure 10 Auscultation of axillae

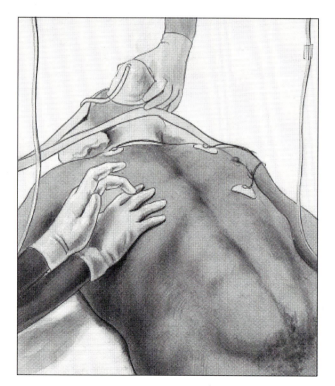

Figure 11 Percussion of chest

The tracheal position, soft tissue deformity and neck vein engorgement should be noted before the cervical collar is put on (Figure 13).

It is important to remember that the upper airway should be the first area to be checked if the patient's ventilation fails or becomes inadequate at any stage of the resuscitation.

TENSION PNEUMOTHORAX

The classical signs of this condition are tachypnoea, tachycardia, hyper-resonance of the hemithorax, shock and, in the late stages, deviation of the trachea (Figure 14). Elevation of the jugular venous pulse does not occur if the patient is hypovolaemic.

If this condition is diagnosed, time should not be wasted in requesting a chest radiograph. Instead, the intrathoracic pressure must be immediately relieved by the insertion of a 14-gauge cannula into the 2nd intercostal space in the mid-clavicular line (Figure 15). A 10 ml syringe is connected to the cannula. If there is a rapid release of air, the diagnosis is confirmed. The cannula is then slid into the intrapleural space and the syringe removed. This manoeuvre transforms a tension pneumothorax into a simple pneumothorax. The clinician now has time to insert a chest drain, which must be accompanied by aggressive fluid resuscitation. The patient's arm is abducted and the 5th intercostal space palpated (Figure 16). Using an aseptic technique, the patient's chest is cleaned and draped (Figure 17).

Local anaesthetic is injected into the 5th intercostal space just anterior to the mid-axillary line (Figure 18). The needle is directed onto the 6th rib and *over its* superior border. This avoids the neurovascular bundle running in the costal groove. A 3 cm transverse incision is made in the anaesthetized area, and extended down to the 6th rib (Figure 19). The pleura *above* the rib is then perforated with a curved clamp and a track is formed (Figure 20).

The clinician then sweeps an extended index finger around the intrapleural space to detect the presence of a ruptured diaphragm or lung adhesions (Figure 21). A fresh incision is made in the mid-axillary line, at either the 4th or 6th intercostal space, if an obstruction is encountered.

A straight clamp is then put over the distal end of the 36-gauge chest drain and the proximal end is inserted into the wound (Figure 22). Directing the tube can be facilitated by a guiding finger or by attaching a straight clamp to the tip of the drain. The tube is connected to either a Portex drainage bag or an underwater drainage set (Figure 23), and the clamp is then removed. Both these systems allow blood and air to the expelled from the thoracic cavity during expiration. The drain is secured with both a purse string suture and tape.

If an underwater drainage set is used, there is initially a rush of air into the container. This settles quickly and the fluid level then simply rises and falls with the respiratory cycle. If this stops, then the chest drain must be checked for obstruction.

CARDIAC TAMPONADE

Cardiac tamponade usually results from a penetrating injury. Direct cardiac damage should be suspected if there are signs of cardiac tamponade (Figure 24) or a wound in the area demonstrated in Figure 25.

Signs of cardiac tamponade
As indicated in Figure 24, these signs are:

(1) Beck's triad, consisting of shock, raised jugular vein pulse, and decreased heart sounds;

(2) Pulsus paradoxus of >10 mmHg; and

(3) Kussmaul's sign (jugular venous pulse elevation on inspiration).

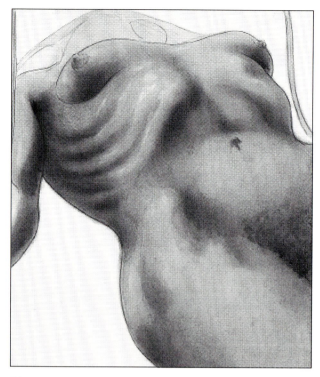

Figure 12 Intercostal indrawing

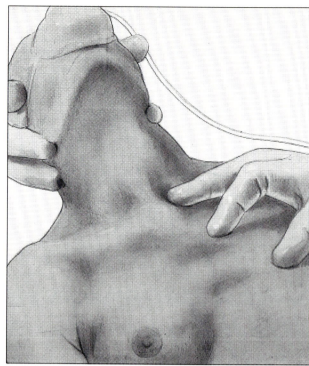

Figure 13 Determination of the position of the trachea

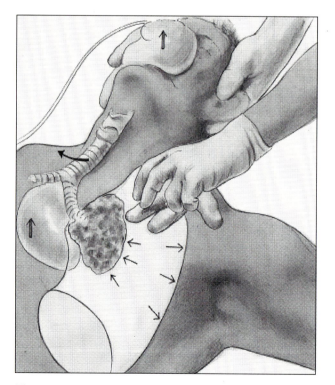

Figure 14 Classical signs of tension pneumothorax

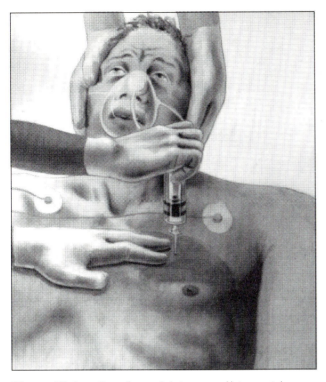

Figure 15 Insertion of cannula into second intercostal space in mid-clavicular line

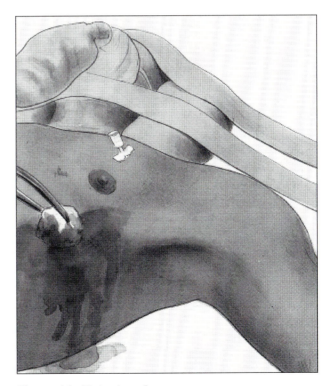

Figure 16 Abduction of arm

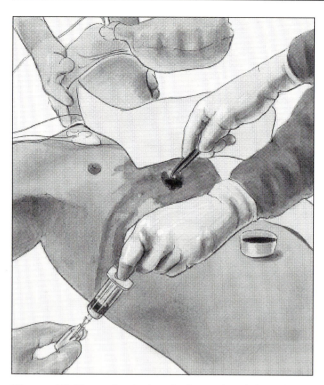

Figure 17 The patient's chest is cleansed and draped

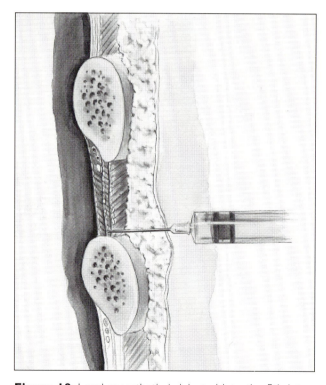

Figure 18 Local anaesthetic is injected into the 5th inter-costal space

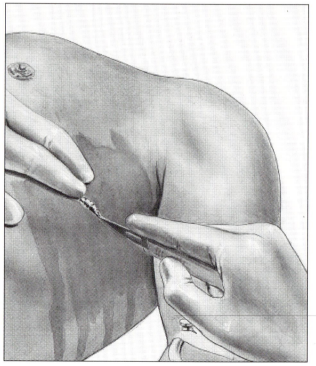

Figure 19 Incision extended down to the 6th rib

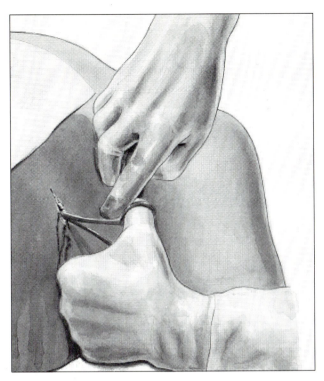

Figure 20 The pleura is perforated with a curved clamp

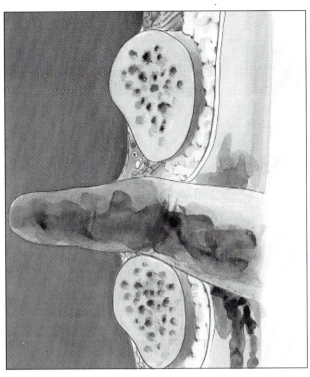

Figure 21 The clinician sweeps an extended index finger around the intrapleural space

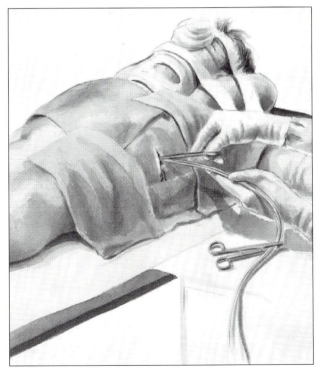

Figure 22 Insertion of tube chest drain with a straight clamp at its distal end

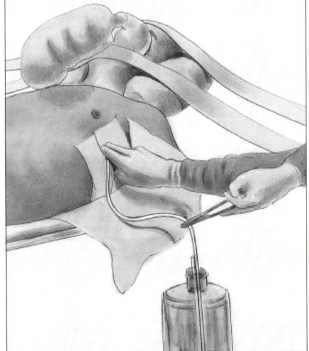

Figure 23 The tube is connected to an underwater set

Unfortunately, only a third of patients with a cardiac tamponade demonstrate these features.

A wound in the area demonstrated

Any wound in the area demonstrated in Figure 25 should cause suspicion of a cardiac tamponade. Emergency treatment consists of increasing the intravenous infusion and aspirating the pericardial sac. The patient is connected to an ECG monitor and the positions of the mediastinum and xiphisternum are noted (Figure 26). If the urgency of the situation allows, the subxiphoid area is cleaned, draped and anaesthetized.

A long, 18-gauge needle, connected to a three-way tap and syringe, is then inserted 1–2 cm inferior to and left of the xiphochondral junction at a 45° angle (Figure 27). Under suction, the needle is advanced towards the tip of the left scapula, *and the ECG continuously monitored* for abnormalities (Figure 28). Upon entering the pericardial sac, the needle is withdrawn and as much unclotted blood as possible is aspirated. The cannula is then left *in situ* and connected to a three-way tap with the stopcock closed.

Dysrhythmias or injury patterns can develop when the tip touches the myocardium. This happens when the needle is pushed too far and as the blood is drained from the pericardium. In these cases, the needle should be slowly withdrawn until a normal ECG tracing is achieved.

Though a needle pericardiocentesis can be lifesaving, a thoracotomy is required in all cases of cardiac tamponade.

OPEN CHEST WOUND

A defect in the chest wall which is greater than two-thirds of the diameter of the trachea will allow air to go preferentially through the hole during inspiration. This causes the lung to collapse (Figure 29).

The immediate treatment is to cover the defect with a dressing sealed only on three sides. This allows air to escape during expiration but none to enter during inspiration (Figure 30). A chest drain should then be inserted in the manner described previously. Surgical closure will be required during the definitive phase.

MASSIVE HAEMOTHORAX

A massive haemothorax occurs either when more than 1.5 litres of blood are found in the hemithorax or when over 200 ml/h are drained following a chest tube insertion. Signs of this condition are a decrease in air entry and dullness to percussion on that side of the chest (Figure 31). The patient is also shocked. The jugular vein pulse may be high or low depending on the degree of hypovolaemia.

A chest drain should be inserted in the manner described previously (Figure 32). These patients will also require type-specific blood, aggressive fluid resuscitation and close observation. If these measures fail, a formal thoracotomy will be needed to stop the bleeding.

FLAIL CHEST

A flail segment occurs when two or more ribs are fractured in two or more places (Figure 33).

Initially there is spasm of the chest wall musculature, leading to rapid, shallow breathing. On palpation of the chest, the grating of broken ribs may be detected. Later, paradoxical movement is seen when the muscles fatigue (Figure 34).

The priority in treating this condition is to correct the hypoxia produced mainly by the underlying pulmonary contusion. High flow, warm, humidified oxygen and adequate resuscitation are needed.

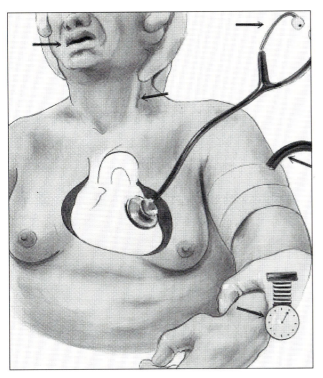

Figure 24 Signs of cardiac tamponade

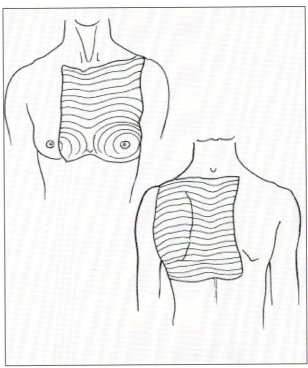

Figure 25 A wound in the shaded area may cause cardiac tamponade

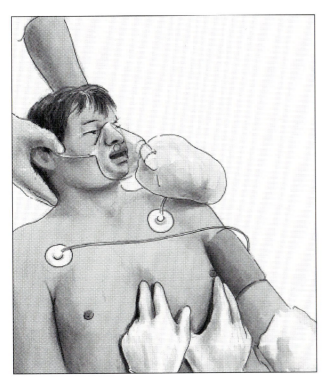

Figure 26 The positions of the mediastinum and xiphisternum are noted

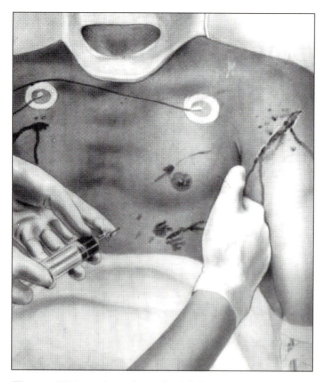

Figure 27 Insertion of needle inferior to and left of the sternocostal angle

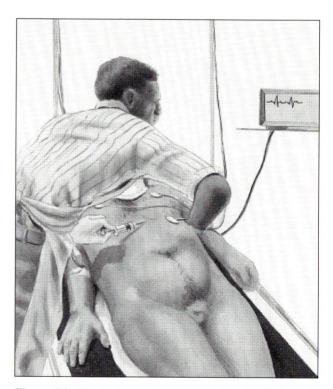

Figure 28 The doctor continuously watches the ECG monitor while performing pericardial aspiration. Under suction, the needle is advanced towards the tip of the left scapula

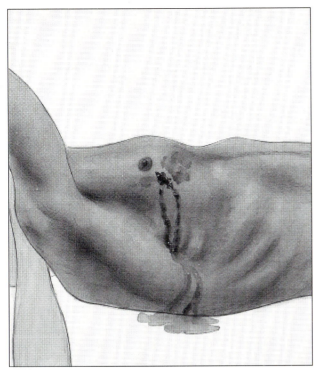

Figure 29 An open chest wound causing the lung to collapse

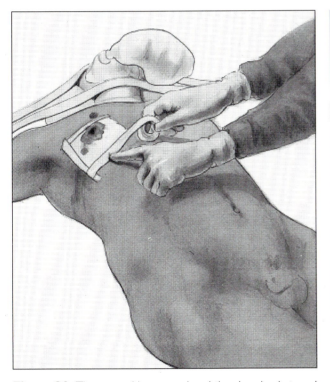

Figure 30 The wound is covered and the dressing is taped on three sides only

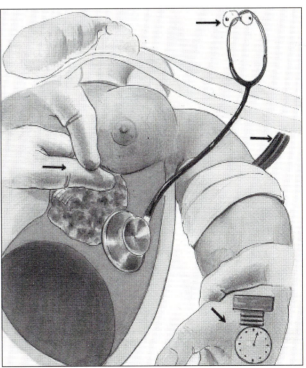

Figure 31 Signs of massive haemothorax

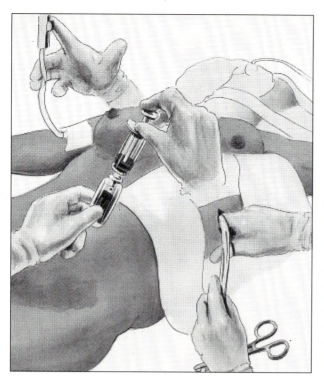

Figure 32 Chest drain insertion in massive haemothorax

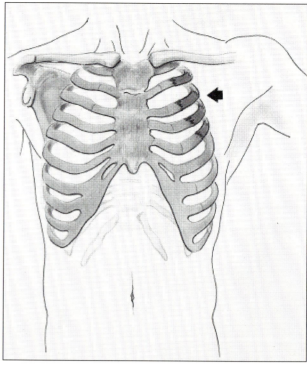

Figure 33 A flail segment

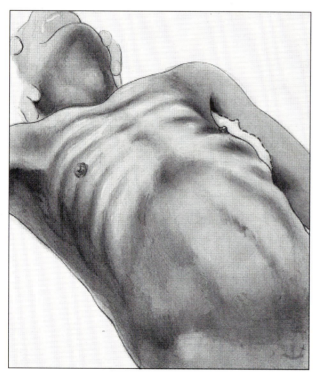

Figure 34 Paradoxical movement

Analgesia, in the form of either an intercostal or epidural block, is carried out during the definitive care phase to facilitate ventilation. A selected group of patients will require artificial, positive pressure ventilation to correct the hypoxia. The conditions for artificial ventilation are:

(1) Falling pO_2 or <60 mmHg on air;

(2) pO_2 <80 mmHg with supplemental oxygen;

(3) Rising pCO_2 or >45 mmHg;

(4) Exhaustion;

(5) Respiratory rate >30/min;

(6) Significant associated injuries of the abdomen and head.

4
Circulation and fluid management

The assessment of the circulatory state is easily over-looked in the patient with multiple injuries. The confused trauma victim is often diagnosed as having a head injury when the primary problem is one of cerebral hypoxia from an airway, breathing or circulatory cause (Figure 1).

CONTROL OF OVERT BLEEDING

Following exclusion of any airway and respiratory problems, the clinician must rapidly control any overt haemorrhage. A clean dressing is applied with pressure and secured with appropriate bandaging if practicable (Figure 2). Direct pressure may be needed until the haemostatic influences of vasoconstriction and coagulation intervene.

Haemostatic forceps, probes and tourniquets are all contraindicated as they can lead to further tissue damage. The only exception is a wound to the scalp which can be responsible for copious blood loss. In this situation, the pressure dressing can be augmented with a self-retaining retractor or temporary sutures (Figure 3). Not infrequently, haemostatic wounds may recommence bleeding once the resuscitation is underway. They should be managed in the manner described above.

ASSESSMENT

The haemodynamic (shock) state of the patient can now be assessed. Shock is defined as inadequate oxygen delivery to vital organs and it can result from several sources (Figures 4–6). This chapter will concentrate on hypovolaemia, which is the commonest cause of shock in the trauma patient, and will briefly mention neurogenic and cardiogenic shock.

Hypovolaemic shock

Intravascular fluid is lost by bleeding, cellular swelling and plasma leakage into the interstitial space (Figure 7). Up to 25% of tissue swelling, following blunt trauma, can be due to plasma leakage.

The body has both neurological and hormonal compensatory mechanisms to maintain adequate tissue oxygenation. These lead to:

(1) A selective decrease in blood flow to less vital organs, such as the skin, muscles, gut and kidneys (Figure 8), as well as an increase in the vascular tone in the venous capacitance vessels. In so doing the venous return to the heart is maximized. Selective vasoconstriction leads to a decrease in urine output and a pale, cold periphery. The former can be measured and the latter tested by using the capillary refill time. In this test,

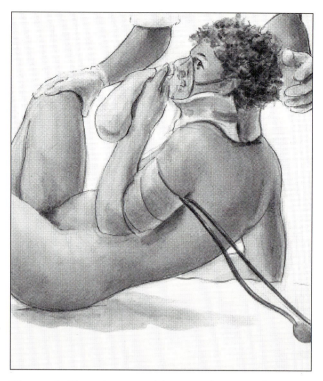

Figure 1 The primary problem may be one of cerebral hypoxia

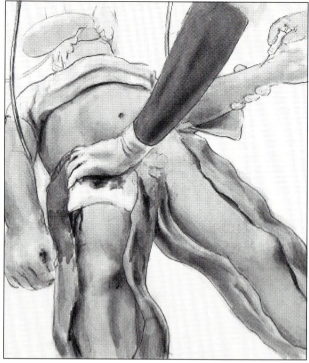

Figure 2 Application of pressure dressing

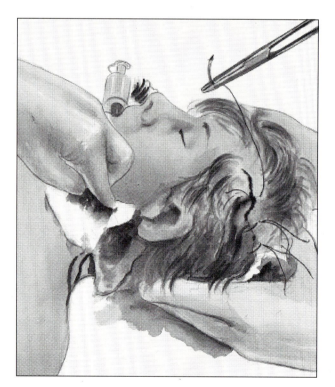

Figure 3 Temporary sutures for a scalp wound

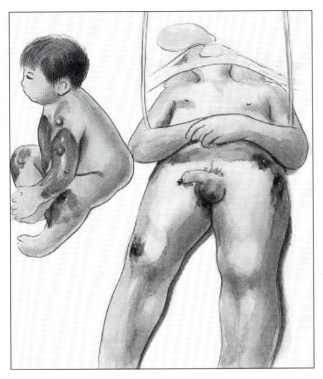

Figure 4 Shock may be caused by hypovolaemia

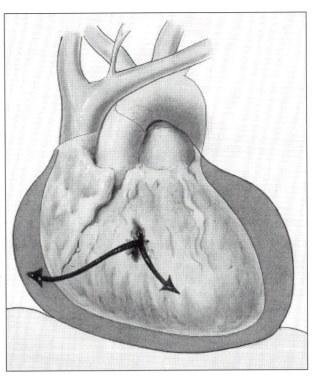

Figure 5 Shock may be caused by inhibition of cardiac output, e.g. cardiac tamponade

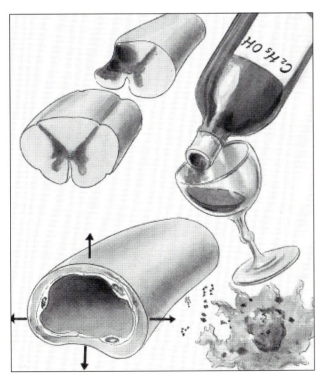

Figure 6 Distributive shock caused by spinal cord injury, septic shock or intoxication leading to dilatation of capacitance and resistance vessels

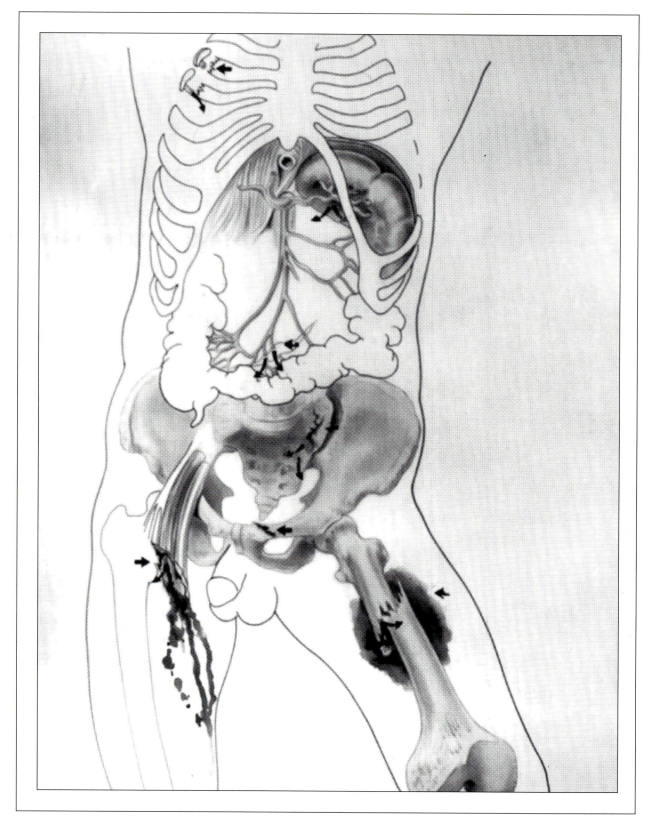

Figure 7 Intravascular fluid loss can be caused by overt bleeding, occult bleeding (pleural space, pelvis, abdomen), haematoma around a fracture, interstitial leak and cellular swelling

the capillary nail bed is blanched by pressure and the time taken for the pink blush to return is recorded (Figure 9). A delay greater than 2 s is abnormal.

(2) A rapid heart rate follows sympathetic and catecholamine stimulation. It is also important to assess the character of the pulse. The reduced stroke volume of the heart that accompanies restriction in the venous return produces a thready pulse. The detection of the pulse in these cases is best achieved by palpation of the carotid (Figure 10) or femoral arteries (Figure 11).

(3) Neurological and hormonal stimulation causes the patient to become agitated. Tachypnoea also occurs but this does not produce any increase in the oxygen content of blood because it is already fully saturated. The metabolic acidosis, resulting from anaerobic metabolism, also stimulates a rise in respiratory rate. The 'clammy' skin, found in shocked patients, is produced by sympathetic stimulation of the sweat glands.

The blood pressure is *not* a sensitive indicator of hypovolaemia. It only falls when the patient's compensatory mechanisms begin to fail. This is usually when 30% of the blood volume has been lost.

Estimating the degree of hypovolaemia

Hypovolaemic shock can be graded into four categories based on the compensatory/decompensatory physical signs described above. The approximate loss of blood volume is given. These are only crude guides but they do highlight the necessity for a full clinical assessment of the patient.

Class 1   The blood volume loss is less than 15% (Figure 12). This is less than 750 ml in the average adult male (normally there is 70 ml of blood per kg of ideal body weight).

Class 2   The blood volume loss is 15–30% (Figure 13). This is between 750 and 1500 ml in the average adult male.

Class 3   The blood volume loss is 30–40% (Figure 14). This is between 1.5 and 2 l in the average adult male.

Class 4   The blood volume loss is over 40% (Figure 15).

Further intravascular volume loss will lead to depression of both the respiratory and heart rate.

Limitations to estimations of blood volume loss

This simple estimation of blood volume loss can produce significant inaccuracies in certain groups of patients.

The elderly patient is sensitive to blood loss. Therefore, volumes smaller than 30% can produce falls in blood pressure. It is also important to remember that the heart rate may be kept artificially low because of a pacemaker or medication (e.g. β-blockers) (Figure 16).

The pulse rate is also dependent upon the individual. An athlete has a larger blood volume and a lower resting pulse than normal (Figure 17). Therefore, (s)he may be demonstrating significant sympathetic stimulation when the heart rate is 80 beats/min.

Pregnancy produces an increase in both blood volume (40–50%) and heart rate (15–20 beats/min), by the third trimester (Figure 18). There is also a fall in blood pressure of 5–15 mmHg during the second trimester.

Hypothermia will reduce the blood pressure, pulse and respiratory rate in its own right, irrespective of any blood loss.

Normal compensation mechanisms can lead to improvements in all the physiological parameters. Consequently, underestimations of blood loss can occur.

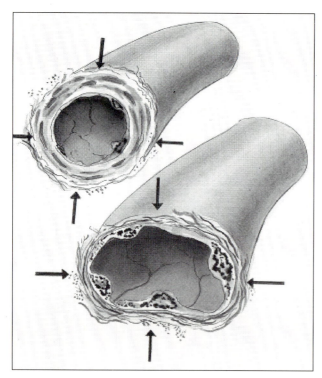

Figure 8 A selective decrease in blood flow to less vital organs

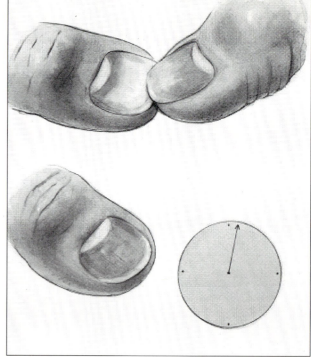

Figure 9 The capillary refill test

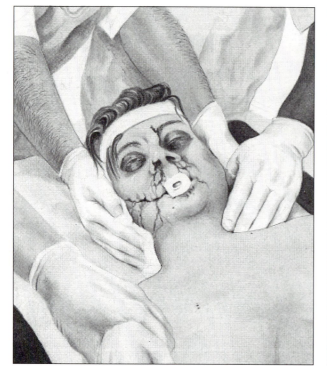

Figure 10 Detection of the pulse by palpation of the carotid artery

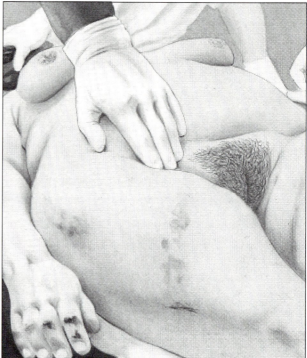

Figure 11 Detection of the pulse by palpation of the femoral artery

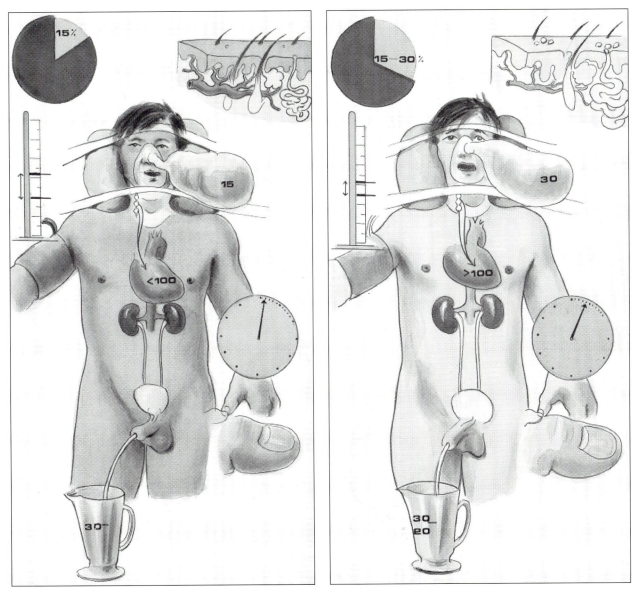

Figure 12 Class 1 of hypovolaemic shock

Figure 13 Class 2 of hypovolaemic shock

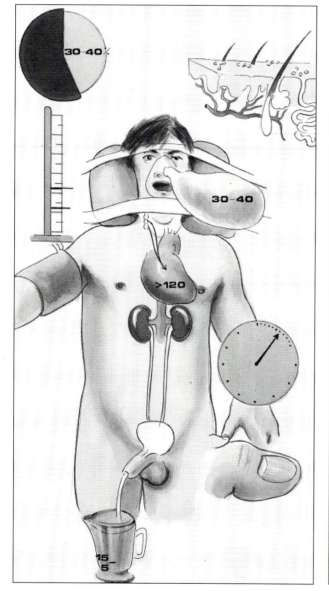

Figure 14 Class 3 of hypovolaemic shock

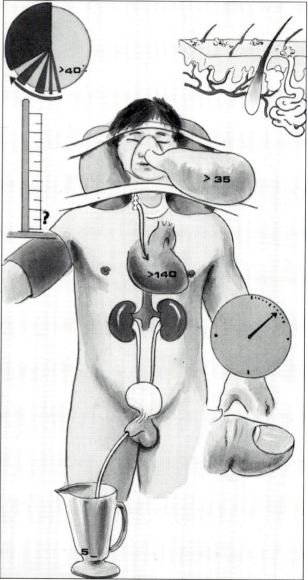

Figure 15 Class 4 of hypovolaemic shock

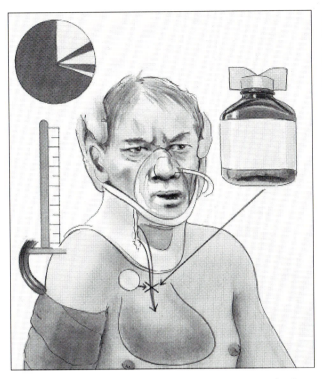

Figure 16 In an elderly patient, the heart rate may be kept artificially low by a pacemaker or medication

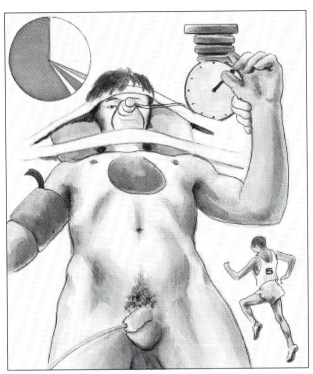

Figure 17 An athlete may demonstrate sympathetic stimulation when his heart rate is 80 beats/min

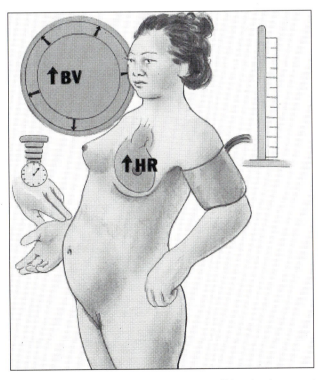

Figure 18 Pregnancy produces increased blood volume and heart rate

RESTORING INTRAVASCULAR VOLUME

It is important to obtain intravenous access as soon as possible so that fluid can be administered. As the bore size and length of the selected cannula controls the rate of infusion, it is recommended that two short, large bore (16 gauge or wider) cannulae are used (Figure 19). This provides a flow rate of 200–300 ml/min. The cannulae are inserted into the antecubital fossa, provided there is no proximal injury. If this is the case, any other available site should be used. Occasionally, the percutaneous venous cannulation is difficult. The patient may be obese, the sites damaged or the veins collapsed due to profound hypovolaemia. In these situations, there are two ways of gaining venous access, venous cutdown or central vein cannulation.

Venous cutdown

Either the medial basilic (Figure 20) or long saphenous veins (Figure 21) are used. After preparation of the skin and, if appropriate, infiltration with local anaesthetic, an incision is made over the vein. Two ligatures are passed; one ligates the distal limb (Figure 22) and the other secures the cannula introduced through the venotomy (Figure 23).

Central vein cannulation

This procedure should *only* be carried out by experienced staff because it has potential for damaging the vein and neighbouring structures.

A Seldinger technique is used to insert a short, wide cannula into either the subclavian or femoral vein. The internal jugular can only be used if a cervical spine injury has been excluded.

After preparation of the skin and, if appropriate, infiltration with local anaesthetic, a needle is inserted into the selected vein (Figure 24). A guide wire is then threaded through the needle and the latter removed (Figure 25). Dilators are then 'rail-roaded' over the guide wire to widen the hole in the vessel (Figure 26). A wide, short cannula can then be slid over the guide wire into the vein and secured in place.

Irrespective of the method used, once the cannula is in place, 20 ml of blood are taken for serum electrolytes, full blood count and blood group and typing. The cannulae are then connected to two 0.5 litre bags of colloid or two 1 litre bags of Hartmann's solution (Figures 27 and 28).

Intraosseous infusion

An intraosseous infusion should be considered, if it is not possible to cannulate a peripheral vein in a child under 5 years. Two sites are possible; one is 3 cm above the lateral epicondyle on the anterior surface of the femur. The other is the anterior surface of the tibia 2–3 cm below the tuberosity (Figure 29). One must use a limb which has no fracture proximal to the infusion site.

The intraosseous needle is inserted at right angles or 60° inferiorly to the perpendicular. There is an obvious give as the needle penetrates the cortex and enters the marrow. The trocar is then removed and the needle aspirated to confirm an adequate position. This should then be sent for the same tests as mentioned above.

The needle is then connected to a normal infusion. Crystalloids run freely into the bone marrow but blood and colloids may need to be put in under pressure.

In adults, the type of fluid chosen, in the initial phase, is of far less importance than the volume of fluid administered. The above solutions must be given rapidly with continuing demand being met with blood. The persistent infusion of non-blood fluids leads to haemodilution with, ultimately, a reduction in oxygen delivery to the tissues. In shocked children, plasma (20 ml/kg) tends to be used rather than crystalloids in the initial phase.

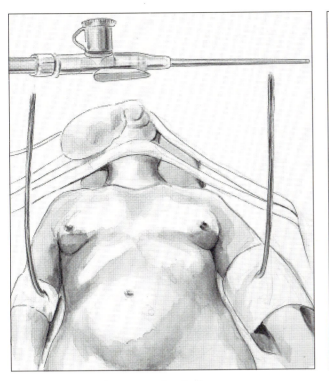

Figure 19 Large bore cannulae for intravenous access

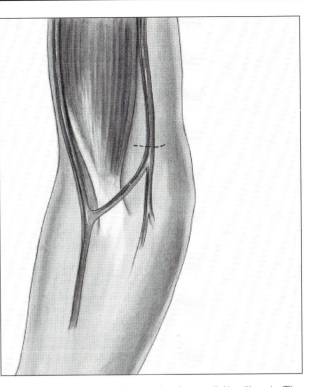

Figure 20 Venous cutdown using the medial basilic vein. The cutdown site is 1 inch laterally from the medial epicondyle

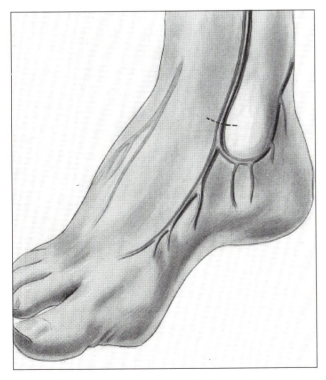

Figure 21 Venous cutdown using the long saphenous veins. The cutdown incision site is 2 inch anteriorly and above the medial malleolus

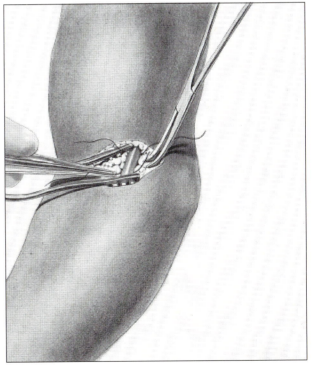

Figure 22 The skin is incised and one ligature ligates the distal vein and the other secures the cannula introduced by venotomy

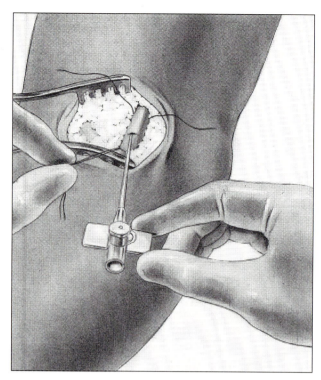

Figure 23 Insertion of cannula into the venotomy

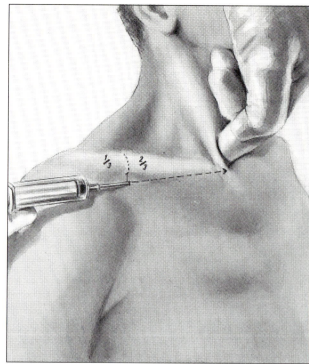

Figure 24 A needle is inserted in the subclavian vein

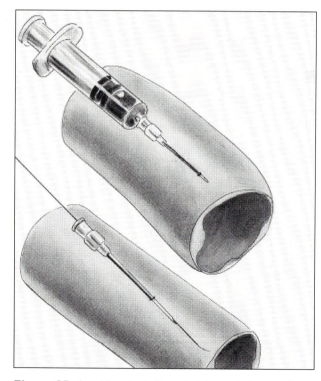

Figure 25 A guide wire is threaded through the needle

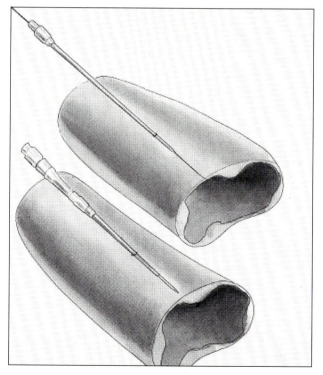

Figure 26 Dilators are rail-roaded over the guide wire

To fully cross-match blood takes over 45 min (Figure 30). Therefore, this should only be requested if the patient can wait that long. Group-specific blood is easier and quicker to process (15 min). This should be used in those patients considered to be in Class 3 shock. Universal donor blood is reserved for Class 4 shock.

Obviously, if fully cross-matched blood has been prepared previously, then this should be used. All fluids given should be warmed before use to prevent iatrogenically induced hypothermia (Figure 31).

REASSESSMENT

It is important to monitor the patient and to measure the vital signs to determine the response to the resuscitation (Figure 32).

Accurate measurement of urine volume will require the insertion of a urinary catheter. The urethra must be inspected for damage, and a rectal examination performed, before perurethral catheterization is carried out in the male patient (see Secondary survey) (Figures 33 and 34).

Accurate monitoring is extremely important in trauma victims with ischaemic heart disease. The early use of invasive monitoring devices, including pulmonary catheters, may be warranted in this type of patient. The assistance from an intensive care clinician should, therefore, be sought early on.

An arterial blood gas sample can be taken at this stage from either radial (Figure 35) or femoral (Figure 15, p. 83) arteries. Metabolic acidosis is invariably the result of anaerobic metabolism in poorly perfused tissues. It should be treated by increasing the ventilation and fluid administration. Sodium bicarbonate is reserved for cases where the pH is less than 7.2.

By the end of the primary survey and resuscitation phase, the estimated blood loss is compared with the patient's response to the volume of fluid provided.

The aim is to achieve adequate organ perfusion. This is indicated by the patient having a urine output greater than 50 ml/h, a normal conscious level and an adequate blood pressure with no tachycardia. There are three options available:

(1) The patient is improving. This implies that the volume loss was less than 20% and that the rate of fluid supply is greater than the rate of bleeding. These patients can wait for a full cross-match but require close observation as they can suddenly deteriorate (Figure 36).

(2) The patient initially improves then deteriorates (Figure 37). This is due to a rapid increase in the rate of bleeding from either a new source developing or a loss of haemostasis at the original site. The majority of these patients require an operation to achieve haemostasis.

(3) The patient does not improve (Figure 38). These patients could be bleeding faster than the rate of supply of fluid, in which case they will require surgery and blood. Dilution of the clotting factors can occur after massive blood loss. The coagulation abnormality must be treated accurately, using regular assessment of the patient's clotting status. Alternatively, this lack of response may be due to shock from a cardiogenic or neurogenic source.

CARDIOGENIC SHOCK

Several conditions can lead to this. Ischaemic heart disease, cardiac contusion and antiarrhythmic drugs can all have negative inotropic effects (Figure 39). The filling of the heart can also be limited by both a tension pneumothorax and a cardiac tamponade (Figure 40). In both cases there is a fall in cardiac output. A tension pneumothorax or cardiac tamponade must be excluded or treated (see Chapter 3). If the source is failure of the heart, then it is essential to discover the trauma victim's past medical history and current medications. Clinically, he may present with evidence of chest trauma, dysrhythmia, a raised jugular venous

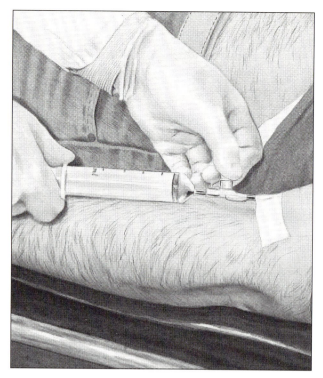

Figure 27 When the cannula is in position, 20 ml of blood is taken

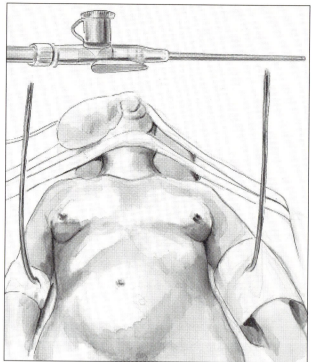

Figure 28 The cannulae are connected to two 0.5 litre bags of colloid or two 1 litre bags of Hartmann's solution

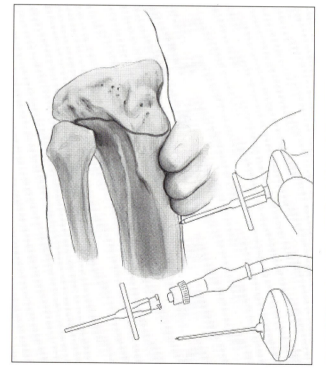

Figure 29 Where intravenous access is difficult, particularly in the young, intraosseous needles permit rapid infusion of fluids. The puncture is made three finger breadths below the tibial tuberosity to avoid damaging epiphyseal growth plate

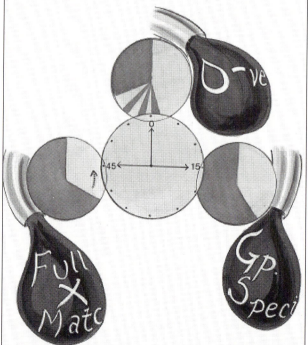

Figure 30 The choice of O-ve, group specific or full cross-match will depend on the immediacy of the transfusion requirement

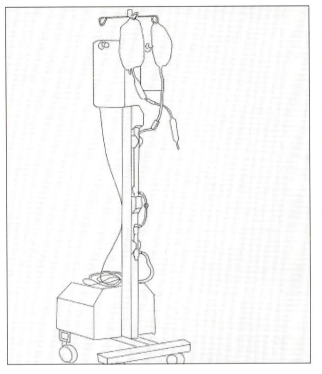

Figure 31 A blood warmer

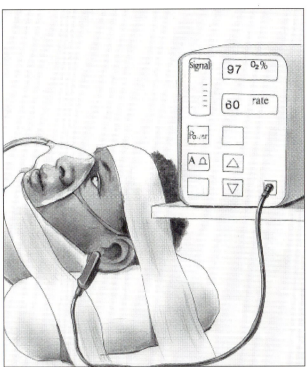

Figure 32 Monitoring with a pulse oximeter

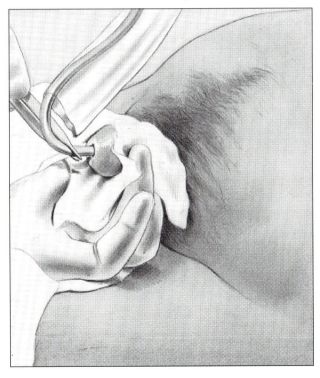

Figure 33 Male catheterization

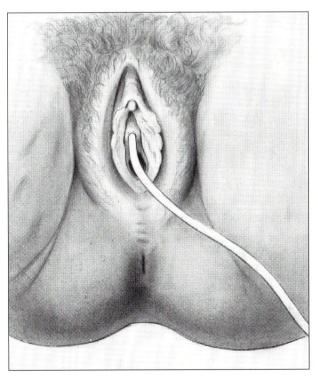

Figure 34 Female catheterization

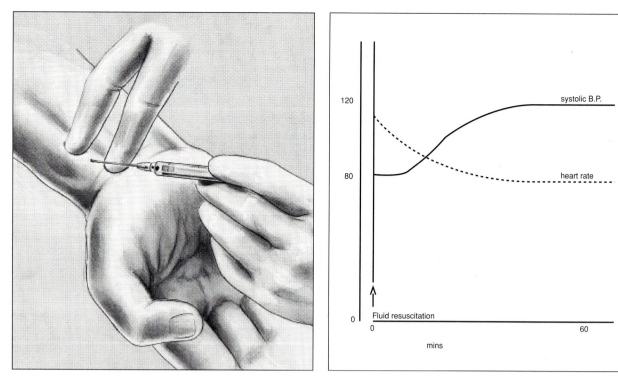

Figure 35 Sampling of arterial blood gas

Figure 36 The patient is improving and can wait for a full cross-match

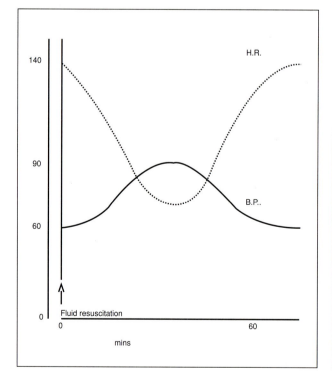

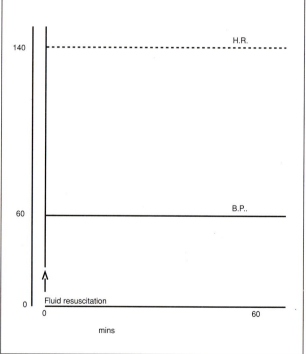
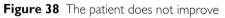

Figure 37 Vital signs improve initially and then deteriorate

Figure 38 The patient does not improve

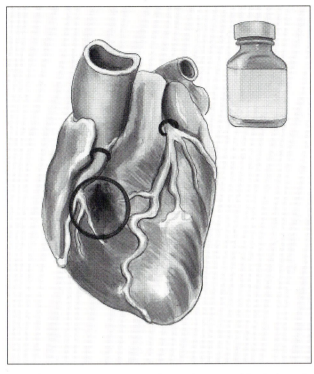

Figure 39 Cardiogenic shock may be caused by ischaemic heart disease, cardiac contusion or antiarrhythmic drugs

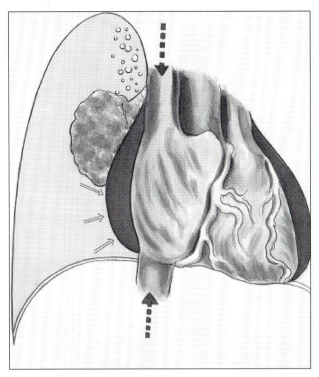

Figure 40 Limited heart filling caused by tension pneumothorax or cardiac tamponade

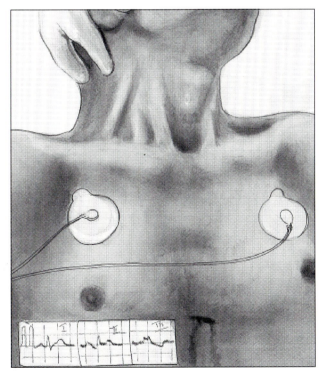

Figure 41 There may be evidence of chest trauma, dysrhythmia, raised jugular vein pulse and signs of shock

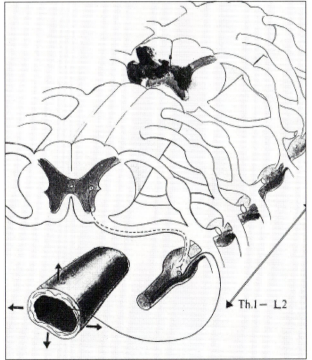

Figure 42 Neurogenic shock will develop if the spinal cord is transected above the level of the sympathetic outflow

pulse and the usual signs of shock (Figure 41). These patients are less able to compensate for hypovolaemia should that co-exist. They require elimination of any hypoxia and invasive monitoring so that the correct amount of fluid is infused. Inotropic and vasodilating drugs may also be required.

NEUROGENIC SHOCK

High spinal injuries eliminate the sympathetic innervation of the vascular system. Generalized vasodilatation occurs, resulting in a fall in cardiac output (Figure 42).

The patient presents with the signs and symptoms of spinal damage, shock and peripheral vasodilation. The tachycardia associated with hypovolaemic shock is not found in this condition because the sympathetic innervation of the heart has been disrupted.

It is important that the correct volume of intravenous fluid is administered to these patients. Too little will not correct the poor tissue perfusion. Too much will produce pulmonary oedema. Therefore, invasive monitoring is required at an early stage in the resuscitation of these trauma victims.

5

Overview and gross dysfunction

Once the assessment and management of the airway, cervical spine, breathing and circulation have been obtained, an overview is taken of the gross neurological dysfunction. This examination has to be swift, therefore the time taken to define accurately the conscious level by the Glasgow Coma Scale is inappropriate during the primary survey. Instead, a simple evaluation of the pupillary reflex and the patient's response to questioning or painful stimuli will ascribe one of the following four labels:

(1) Alert, oriented and co-operating with the examiner;

(2) Eyes opening to verbal command;

(3) Movement in an attempt to remove a painful stimulus;

(4) Unresponsive to any stimulus.

Although each category contains a spectrum of cerebral dysfunction, accurate definition into a group is possible and transition from one group to another is highly significant. Should there be any deterioration, the clinician must first reassess the patient's airway, ventilation and circulatory status before considering an intracranial cause.

The opening enquiry, 'What happened?', invites the alert patient to recount what he has experienced, and so demonstrate adequate cerebral perfusion (Figure 1).

The patient who only opens his eyes to commands usually speaks in a confused manner and can be abusive (Figure 2). Alcohol or drug intoxication can make assessment difficult; however, evidence for its consumption should not distract the examiner. Too often, drunk trauma victims receive suboptimal management because neurological signs are attributed to alcohol intoxication.

The application of painful stimuli is only required if there is no response to vocal commands (Figure 3). Starting with a light pressure over the supratrochlear nerve or nail bed, the magnitude is increased until a response is elicited. Patients with a markedly depressed consciousness require a fairly painful stimulus to produce arousal. However, the force applied must always fall short of that which would produce tissue damage and obviously areas of trauma must be avoided.

The final group includes those patients who are either unresponsive (Figure 4) or produce a decerebrate or decorticate posture to a painful stimulus (Figures 5 and 6). Brain damage of this severity may be suspected from the external appearance of the head and pupil status. It is important to remember that the patient will be unresponsive if (s)he has been pharmacologically paralysed or if there is significant neurological disruption. Once the A, B and Cs have been completed, these patients will require a computed tomography scan.

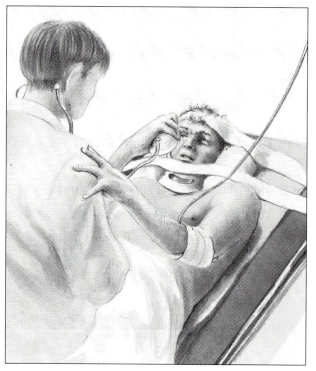

Figure 1 The patient is alert, oriented and co-operates with the examiner

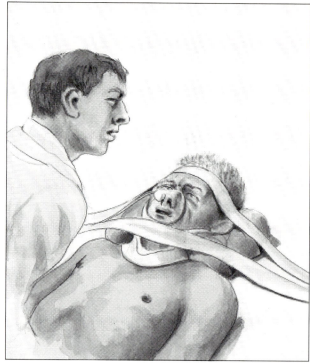

Figure 2 The patient responds to verbal command

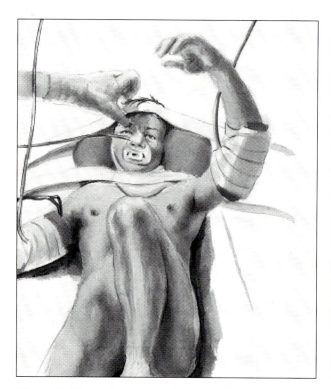

Figure 3 The patient responds to a painful stimulus

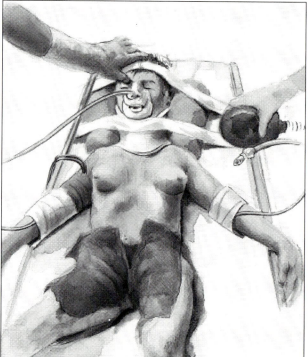

Figure 4 The patient is unresponsive to stimulus

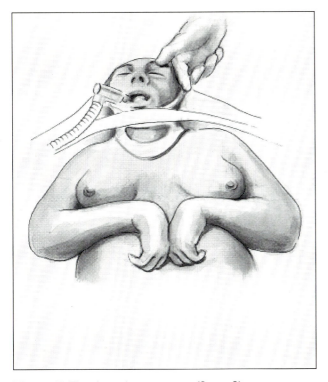

Figure 5 The decorticate posture (Score 3)

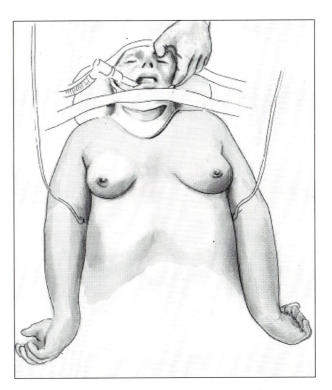

Figure 6 The decerebrate/extension to pain posture (Score 2)

6
Exposure and essential medication

EXPOSURE

Exposure of the patient must be complete in any case of major trauma so that *all* the injuries can be assessed (Figure 1). The possibility of spinal injuries means that garments cannot simply be slid off; instead all clothing must be cut along the seams. Considerable care should be taken because of the possible underlying tissue damage.

Initially, the neck, chest and upper limbs are exposed to facilitate the first three parts of trauma care – namely airway and cervical spine control, breathing and circulation (Figure 2). Once this has been completed, one of the team can remove the remaining clothes (Figure 3).

Large scissors are usually effective in achieving swift but careful removal of even motorcycle leatherwear. Cutting along the seams allows the material to fall away from the body. Clothing is eventually completely removed at the end of the secondary survey when the patient can be moved in a coordinated fashion.

Careful log rolling of the patient enables the patient's back to be exposed without jeopardizing the spinal cord (Figure 4). Three team members are required to turn the patient under the command of a fourth person who stabilizes the patient's head and neck (Figure 5). A vertical lift, with adequate numbers of staff, under the command of the neck supporter, will also enable clothing to be cleared and the back exposed (Figure 6).

Whichever method is used, the team leader should then examine the back thoroughly for overt and occult injuries. All debris is carefully removed as it may contain glass. Any open wound should be covered with a sterile dressing to prevent further contamination (Figure 7).

Clothing that is penetrating a wound with other foreign material should be removed in the operating theatre (Figure 8). Torrential haemorrhage or significant contamination may follow its inopportune extraction.

The pneumatic antishock garment (PASG) may have been put on the patient, and inflated, by the prehospital personnel to maintain venous return to the hypovolaemic patient (Figure 9). This garment must be removed in a controlled manner so that a sudden collapse in the venous return to the haemodynamically unstable patient is prevented (Figure 10). Therefore, before the PASG is deflated, the patient *must* have:

(1) Two intravenous lines in place with fluid being infused;

(2) Vital signs accurately and continuously monitored;

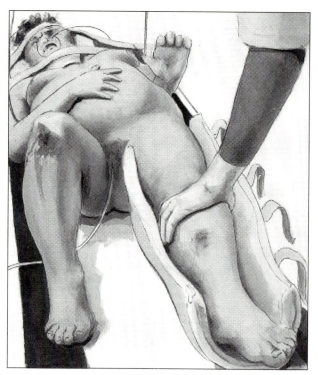

Figure 1 Exposure of the patient must be complete in any case of major trauma

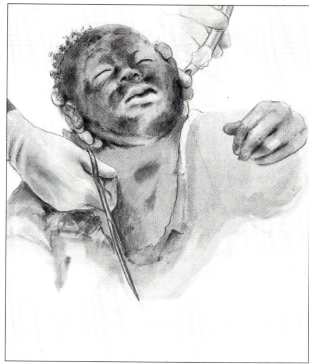

Figure 2 Exposure of neck, chest and upper limbs

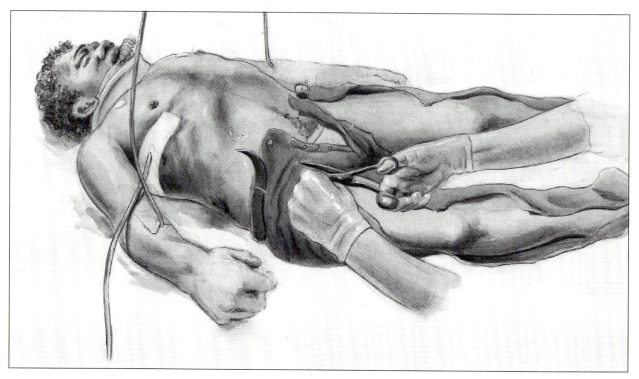

Figure 3 Removal of remaining clothes

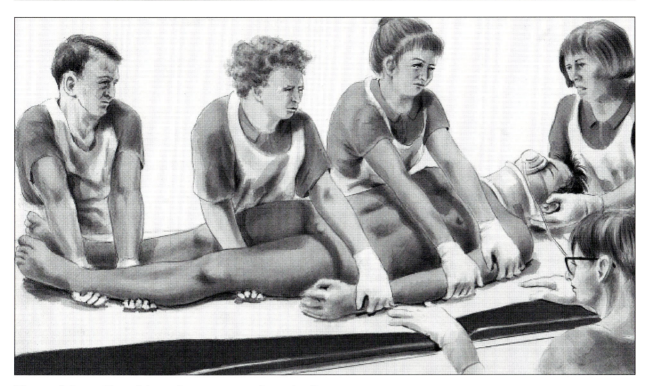

Figure 4 Log rolling of the patient to expose the patient's back

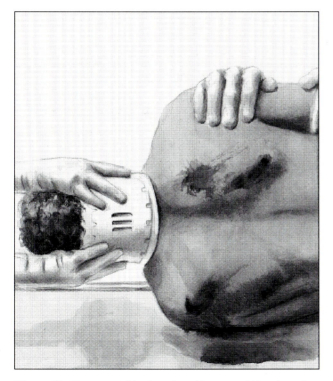

Figure 5 Close-up of the hand position to stabilize the spine during the turn

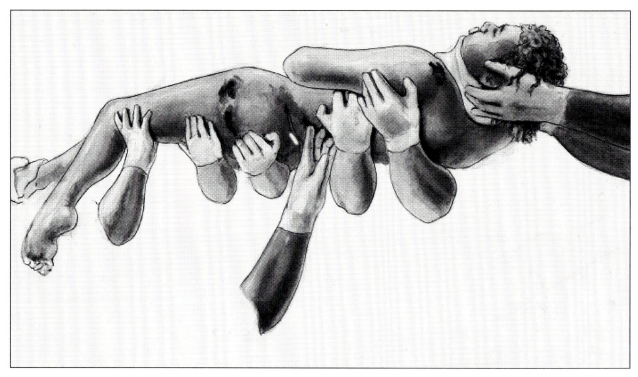

Figure 6 The vertical lift

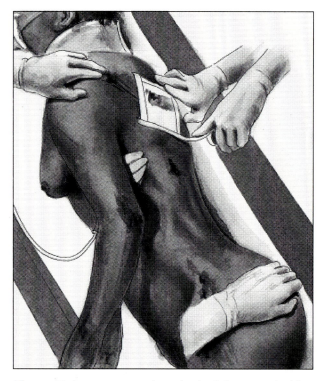

Figure 7 An open wound on the back is covered with a sterile dressing

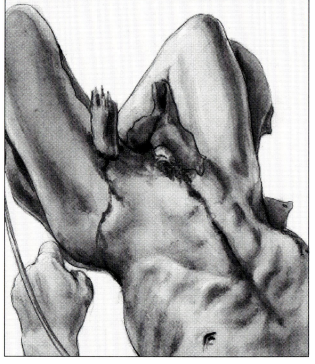

Figure 8 Clothing that is penetrating a wound should be removed in the operating theatre

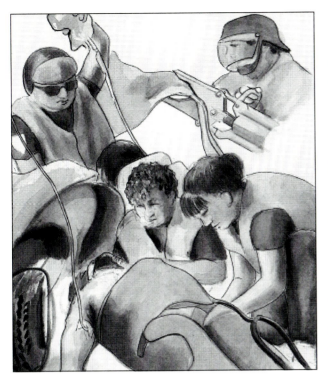

Figure 9 The pneumatic antishock garment in place

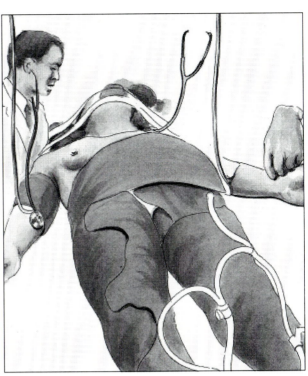

Figure 10 This garment must be removed in a controlled manner

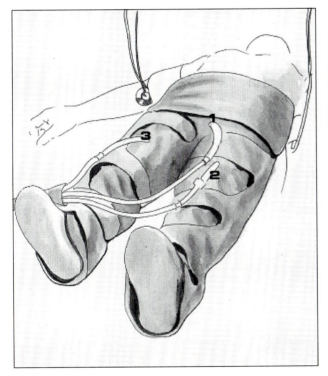

Figure 11 The order of deflation of the antishock garment

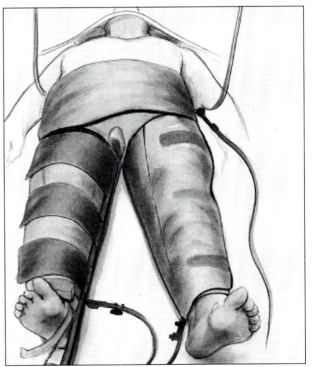

Figure 12 A splint is best left initially *in situ*

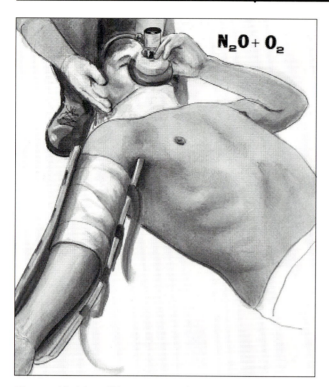

Figure 13 Use of Entonox as a short-term analgesic agent

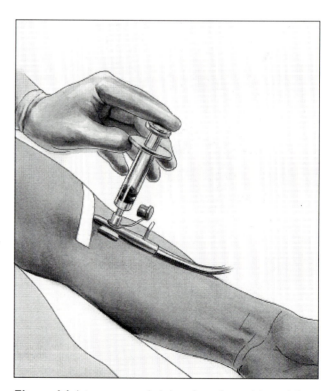

Figure 14 Intravenous administration of morphine sulphate and metoclopramide

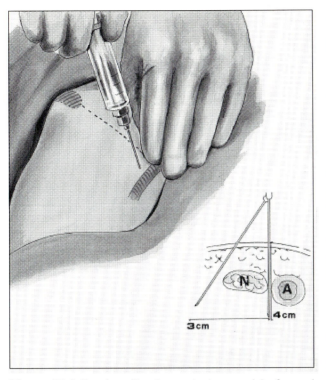

Figure 15 Infiltration of local anaesthetic around the femoral nerve showing the depth and extent of infiltration

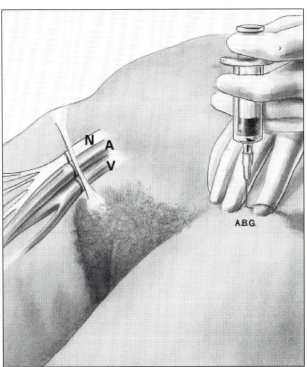

Figure 16 Anatomy within the femoral triangle: neuro-vascular structures from medial to lateral proceed vein, artery, nerve. Obtaining an arterial blood gas sample

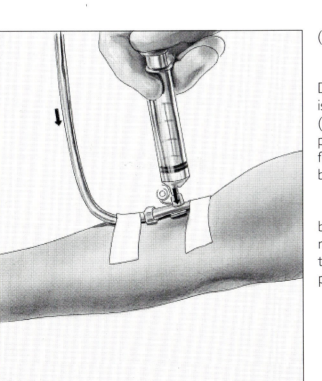

Figure 17 Intravenous administration of broad-spectrum antibiotics by infusion or slow injection

(3) Haemodynamic stability or be in an operating theatre with a prepared surgical team.

Deflation is carried out slowly – the abdominal section is deflated first, followed by each leg section in turn (Figure 11). The procedure must be halted if the blood pressure falls by more than 5 mmHg at any stage. The fluid infusion should then be accelerated until the blood pressure is restored.

Along similar lines, previously applied splints are best left initially *in situ*, as they minimize fracture movement, blood loss, pain and wound contamination (Figure 12). The analgesic requirements of the patient are therefore reduced.

Table I Tetanus immunization in adults

Active regime
0.5 ml adsorbed tetanus toxoid. The 1st dose is followed by a 2nd dose after 6–8 weeks, a third dose after a further
4–6 months, and a booster dose every 10 years

Status regarding wounds
If the fully active regime was administered more than 5 years but less than 10 years previously, 0.5 ml of toxoid is
given for *tetanus-prone* wounds

If the patient is of partial active status (i.e. he received two or more doses of toxoid more than 10 years previously),
he is given 0.5 ml of toxoid for *all* wounds

Uncertain status
0.5 ml toxoid for non-tetanus prone wounds
0.5 ml toxoid + 250 units of human tetanus immune globulin for tetanus-prone wounds

ESSENTIAL MEDICATION

Once the primary survey and resuscitation phase have been completed, consideration of essential medications can be made. These include analgesic requirements, and tetanus and antibiotic prophylaxis.

Analgesic requirements

Injuries are often extremely painful, especially when they are associated with limb fractures. Good communication, gentle handling and correct fracture immobilization are all very effective in reducing pain. However, other agents may be required.

Entonox is an effective short-term analgesic agent, for example during splintage (Figure 13).

Morphine sulphate (diluted to 1 mg/ml) can be used for more severe cases. It is given in small intravenous increments until the patient's pain is relieved. The patient must be continuously monitored for developing respiratory depression, confusion and analgesic effect. Intravenous metoclopramide should be given at the same time to reduce the chances of vomiting (Figure 14).

Regional analgesia can be very effective in cases of limb trauma (Figures 15 and 16).

Tetanus prophylaxis

Tetanus prophylaxis must be provided in all patients who have a tetanus-prone wound (Table 1).

Antibiotic prophylaxis

Broad-spectrum antibiotics are often given in cases of compound fractures to help reduce the chances of infection. These must be given intravenously and in accordance with the departmental protocol (Figure 17).

7

Blood and radiological investigations relevant to the patient with multiple injuries

BLOOD INVESTIGATIONS

During the rapid initial phase of the resuscitation, certain vital investigations are carried out.

The request for grouping and cross-matching blood on the clotted specimen taken is the priority investigation (Figure 1). When a number of unidentified patients have to be dealt with, it is wise to establish a code for each. Labelling of the patient and specimen prevents confusion in handling results. If additional blood is taken, specimens can be saved and labelled for later analysis, for example, samples for electrolyte, haemoglobin, alcohol and drug screens.

RADIOLOGICAL INVESTIGATIONS

A lateral cervical, chest and anterior-posterior pelvic radiographs should be taken in all cases of blunt trauma.

Lead protective aprons should therefore be available for members of the trauma team who need to attend to the patient during radiographic exposure.

The cervical spine lateral view

This view excludes 85% of cervical spine injuries. All seven vertebrae in the neck need to be visualized from the atlas to the top of the 1st thoracic vertebra. The caudal bones are frequently obscured by the shoulders but traction distally on undamaged upper limbs will often uncover them. If this fails, a swimmer's view can be taken lifting the arm as shown (Figure 2). If upper limb movements are prohibited a supine oblique projection will visualize the cervico-thoracic region.

The clinician must have a systematic approach when studying the radiographs.

(1) Initially the full complement of cervical vertebrae are counted and the top of T1 established.

(2) The four longitudinal contours are checked (Figure 3). Lines 1 and 2 are the anterior and posterior longitudinal lines of the vertebral bodies. Line 3 is the spinolaminar line marking the posterior margin of the spinal canal, which dilates slightly at C2. Line 4 consists of the smooth contour of the tips of the spinous processes.

(3) The soft tissue shadows are inspected (Figure 4). The normal appearance features the prevertebral shadow formed by the muscles of the pharynx and the ligaments anterior to the vertebrae. The air in the pharynx appears black. At the level of the cricoid ring (which is also detectable), this shadow is thickened by the oesophagus to an upper limit of 22 mm instead of 7 mm above.

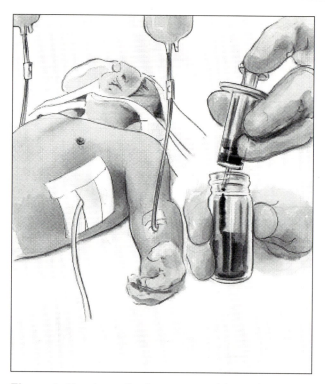

Figure 1 Blood sampling for cross-matching and additional analysis

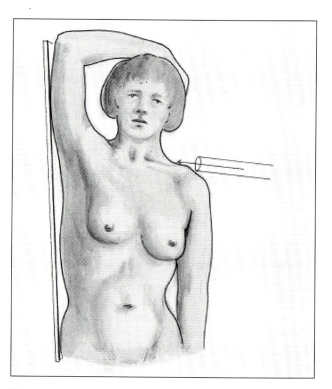

Figure 2 The swimmer's view X-ray

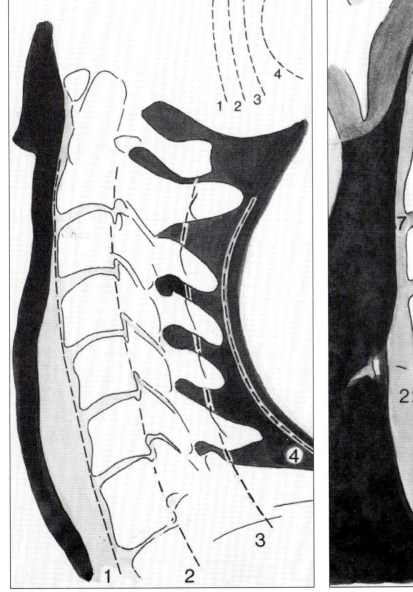

Figure 3 The four longitudinal contours

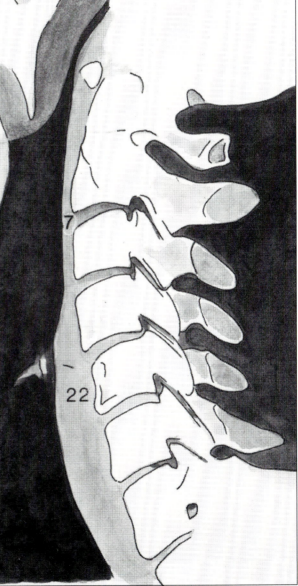

Figure 4 Cervical soft tissue shadows. The maximum thickness of the prevertebral shadow is shown in mm

Thickening of this image from haematoma may be the only radiographic indicator of severe injury. Blood may track down from maxillo-facial trauma into this region.

(4) Each element is then analysed in turn – vertebral bodies, lateral mass, pedicles and facet joints, laminae and the spinous processes.

The spinal ligaments contribute greatly to the stability of the cervical spine. The anterior longitudinal ligament checks hyperextension. The facet joints in combination with their ligaments and the interspinous ligaments prevent excessive flexion.

Radiographs must be studied for the signs of instability (Figure 5). These are:

(1) An angulation of over 10° between vertebral bodies;

(2) Fanning of the spinous processes;

(3) Facet joint overriding;

(4) Facet joint widening;

(5) More than 3.5 mm displacement forwards of one vertebra to another;

(6) Compression fracture of more than 25% in height of the vertebral body.

The proximal two vertebrae and the skull have a greater degree of freedom relative to the rest of the cervical spine. Virtually all the stability in this region is conferred by the ligaments. The alar and cruciform ligaments are shown in Figures 6 and 7. The transverse ligament maintaining the atlanto-axial articulation is also seen in Figure 7. Rupture of this structure allows dorsal displacement of the odontoid peg detectable on the lateral film. Frequently, fatal cord damage accompanies disruption of these ligaments.

Equivocal C1 and C2 fractures on the lateral film may be confirmed with a 'through-the-mouth' view. The image of the posterior arch of C1, the occiput or the teeth can be mistaken for this fracture when their images overlie the dens of C2 (Figure 8). True fractures of the dens are demonstrated in the lower part of Figure 8. In children, this site is marked by an epiphysis.

The Jefferson burst fracture of C1 can also be seen on this view (Figure 9). It produces the displacement laterally of the facet of C1 relative to C2 and is unstable (Figure 10). It is produced by striking the top of the head, as for example when diving into a shallow pool. Other compression forces produce burst fractures of the vertebral bodies.

Examples of hyperextension injuries are given (Figure 11). The hangman's fracture represents a fracture of the pars interarticularis of C2. This can be seen on a lateral X-ray. Rupture of the anterior longitudinal ligament, accompanied by an avulsion fracture, is seen in other gross hyperextension injuries to the cervical spine.

Predominantly flexion forces are responsible for the markedly unstable 'teardrop' fracture and ligament disruption (Figure 12). Angulation forwards and displacement can occur and further insult to the spinal cord is seen with retropulsion of the posterior fragment of the vertebral body.

Additional rotational forces at injury are responsible for dislocation of one or both facet joints (Figure 13). Bifacetal dislocation has forward displacement of over half a vertebral body. Unifacetal dislocation produces less anterior displacement and a rotational deformity seen on the lateral film.

Radiographs of the chest

The normal anterior-posterior chest film exhibits magnification of the cardiac shadow and mediastinal structures (Figure 14). The diaphragm is also higher than the more familiar erect posterior-anterior exposure. The supine film will not show sharp fluid–gas

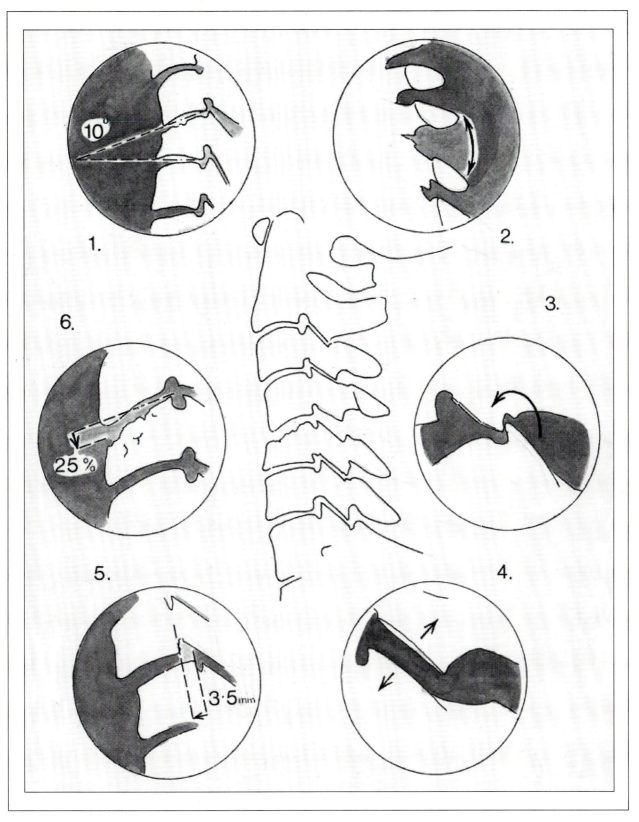

Figure 5 Signs of cervical instability

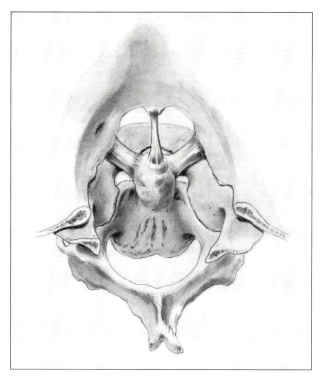

Figure 6 The alar ligaments

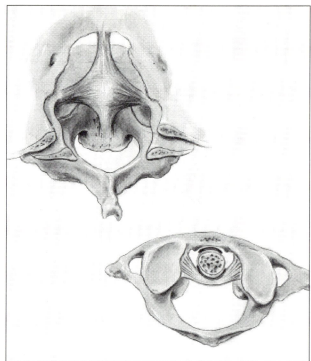

Figure 7 The upper diagram shows the cruciform ligament and the lower diagram is of the transverse ligament of the atlas with the dens seen in cross-section

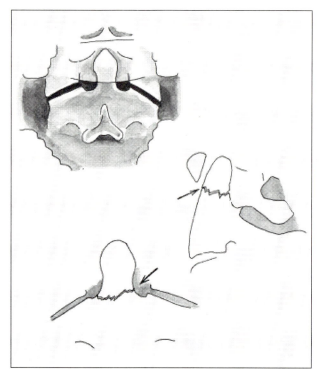

Figure 8 A 'through-the-mouth' view with the normal shadow overlying the dens. True fractures of the dens can be seen on the anterior-posterior and lateral views, arrowed on the diagram

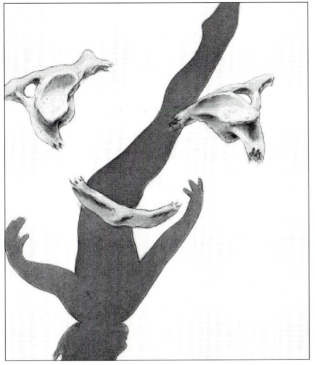

Figure 9 A Jefferson burst fracture of C1, a common diving injury

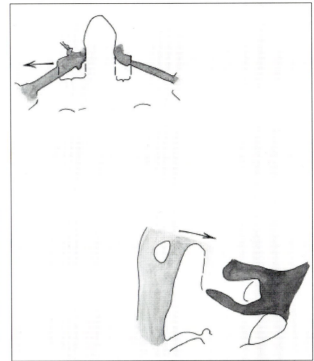

Figure 10 The upper diagram shows the Jefferson burst fracture with displacement. The lower diagram demonstrates the ligamentous disruption with the posterior displacement of the C2 vertebra

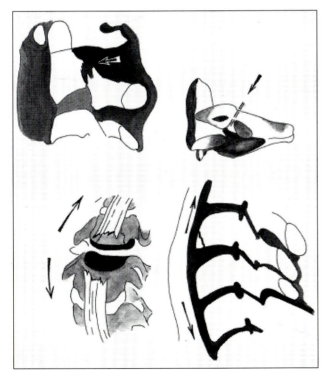

Figure 11 Hyperextension injuries: top left, hangman's fracture; top right, demonstrating the pars interarticularis; bottom left, rupture of the anterior longitudinal ligament; bottom right, avulsion fracture from the vertebral body

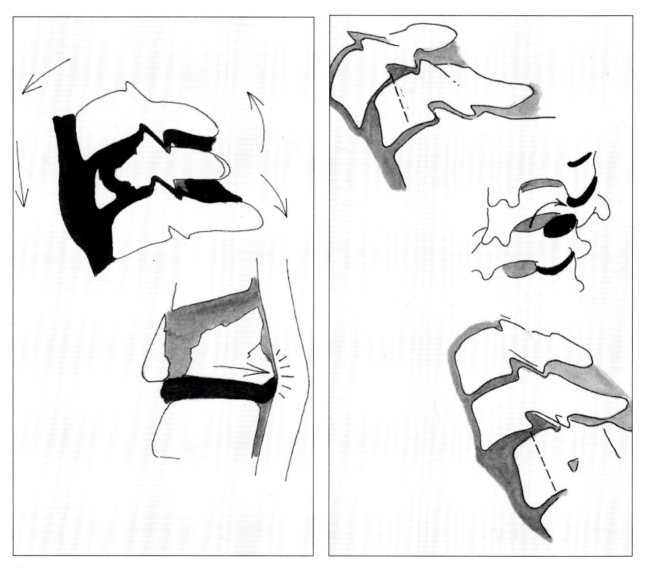

Figure 12 Top, 'teardrop' fracture; bottom, retropulsion of a fragment impinging on the spinal cord

Figure 13 Top, bifacetal dislocation; middle, oblique view of overriding facet; bottom, unifacetal dislocation

levels or gas beneath the diaphragm. The edges of the scapulae frequently intrude onto the lung fields and the glenohumeral joints and the root of the neck are noted. Scrutiny should follow a systematic approach, including inspection of soft tissues and bones as well as thoracic structures.

Radiological signs of potentially life-threatening conditions

(1) *Pulmonary contusion* Rib fractures are not necessary for lung contusion to occur.

(2) *Ruptured diaphragm* (Figure 15) This is more common on the left side. The 'raised hemi-diaphragm' appearance is produced by abdominal viscera herniating through a rent in the diaphragm. A nasogastric tube may highlight the defect. This diagnosis is often missed. Fractured lower ribs raise suspicion of this diagnosis and possible ruptured liver or spleen.

(3) *Dissecting thoracic aorta* (Figure 16) Rupture of the aorta causes haemorrhage and widening of the mediastinum with loss of the normal aortic knuckle. Tracking of the blood also produces capping of the lung fields and associated haemothorax.

(4) *Airway rupture* A significant force is needed to rupture a major vessel or bronchus. Fractures of the upper three ribs may be present. Pneumo-mediastinum and extensive surgical emphysema are seen. A persistent pneumothorax, despite effective chest drainage, is highly suggestive of the diagnosis.

(5) *Oesophageal rupture* Oesophageal rupture, like airway rupture, may have no radiological signs or later a pneumomediastinum may develop.

Immediate life-threatening thoracic conditions

Immediate life-threatening thoracic conditions usually present with dramatic physical signs and, consequently, life-saving measures can and should be started before a chest X-ray is taken.

The six conditions are:

(1) *Respiratory obstruction* The object may be seen with distal collapse of the obstructed lung segment.

(2) *Tension pneumothorax* (Figure 17) The affected lung is completely collapsed. The high pressure in the pleural space displaces the heart and mediastinum, deviates the trachea and flattens the diaphragm.

(3) *Massive haemothorax* (Figure 18) Blood pools collect in the pleural space behind and inferior to the lung. A 'white out' appearance is seen.

(4) *Cardiac tamponade* (Figure 19) The quantity of blood in the pericardial sac required to compromise heart function is not large. The increased cardiac shadow may not be an impressive feature.

(5) *Flail chest* The lung field demonstrates multiple rib fractures with potential for a free-moving segment. This degree of injury is associated with significant underlying pulmonary contusion. The fluffy radiological signs develop within 6 h.

(6) An *open chest* wound will produce a pneumothorax on the affected side. Large defects will reduce ventilation of the other lung.

Pelvis anterior-posterior radiograph

Disruption of the pelvic ring is associated with extensive haemorrhage from the fractures themselves and also the lacerated pelvic veins (Figure 20).

An anterior-posterior radiograph is taken to confirm this fracture of the pelvis. Management is influenced as follows. Estimates of the blood lost and fluid requirements are markedly increased. The application of a pelvic external fixator is considered. This stabilizes the bleeding vessels, allowing haemostasis to occur.

Diligent examination will reveal whether the ring structure of the pelvis is broken. The sacroiliac joints

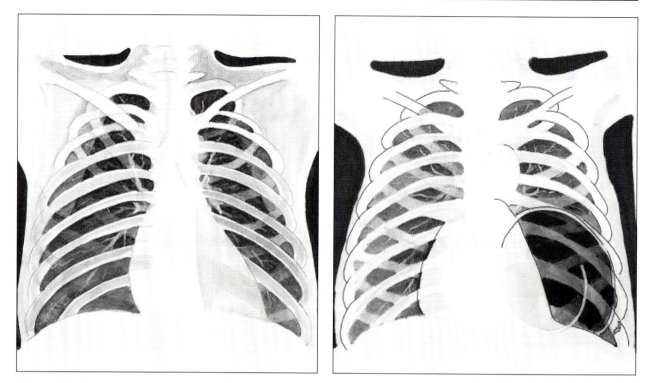

Figure 14 The normal anterior-posterior chest radiograph

Figure 15 Radiograph of ruptured left hemidiaphragm, gastric air bubble lying in chest cavity with nasogastric tube in place

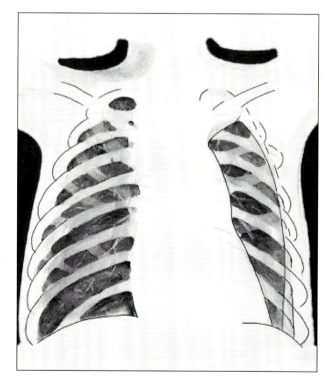

Figure 16 Radiograph of dissecting thoracic aorta with widening of the upper mediastinum and capping of left lung field with associated haemothorax

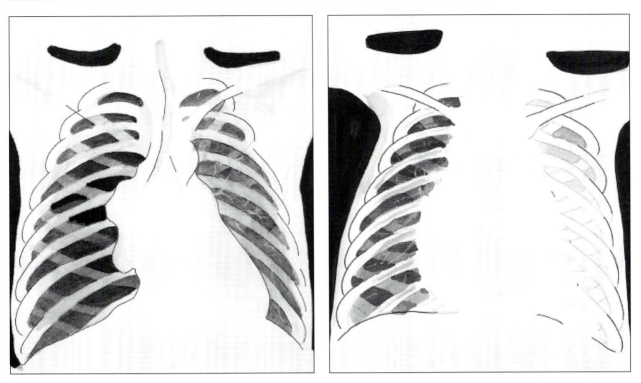

Figure 17 Tension pneumothorax with complete right lung collapse and displacement of trachea and mediastinal structures

Figure 18 Massive haemothorax with white-out of lung field from blood in thoracic cavity

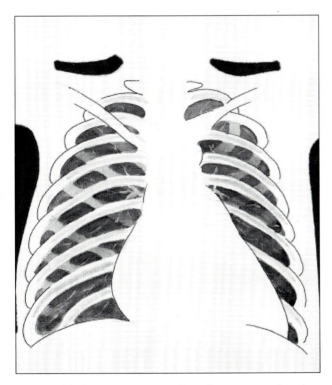

Figure 19 Late appearance of cardiac tamponade when pericardial enlargement occurs. Frequently, the chest X-ray will appear normal

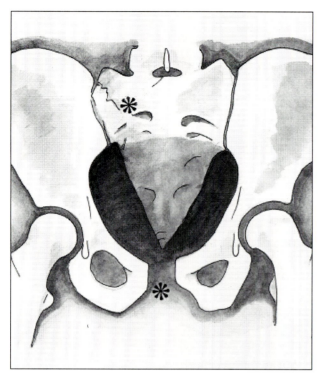

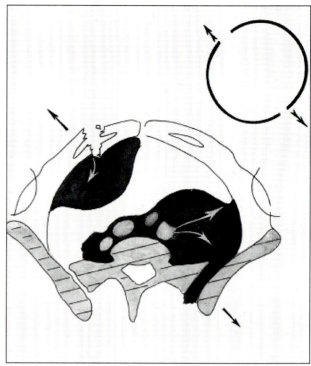

Figure 20 Anterior-posterior view of the pelvis with ring disruption. Symphyseal disruption and fracture of the wing of the sacrum are marked

Figure 21 This is a view looking down onto a pelvic ring, which is disrupted. The fracture line runs through the sacro-iliac joint and pubic rami with attendant haemorrhage from pelvic veins

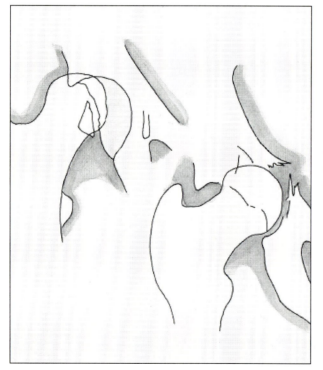

Figure 22 Left, posterior dislocation of the hip joint; right, fracture of the acetabulum

may be dislocated and the pubic rami fractured. Separation of the symphysis may be associated with fracture of the ilium or sacrum. Interruption of the sacral foramenal lines indicates fracture of the sacrum (Figure 21).

The plain pelvic film also reveals hip joint pathology, for example dislocation of the hip or fracture of the acetabulum (Figure 22). Pelvic arch fractures are often coupled with significant injury to the bladder or urethra.

8

Secondary survey

The secondary survey consists of a detailed head-to-toe assessment of the *whole* patient. The objective is to detect all the patient's injuries so that a correct management plan can be devised. Nevertheless, should the patient deteriorate at any stage, the clinician must reassess the patient using the A, B, C protocol described in the primary assessment.

HEAD AND NECK

Scalp
The whole of the scalp needs to be examined for lacerations, swellings or depressions (Figure 1). This is carried out in a front-to-back fashion; however, the occiput will have to wait until the patient is turned or the cervical spine cleared radiologically and clinically. Each wound must be visually inspected (Figure 2) with scalp haemorrhage controlled by either digital pressure or a self-retaining retractor.

Neurological state
This is carried out by assessing three parameters: consciousness level; pupillary response; lateralizing signs. These parameters need to be continuously measured during the patient's stay in the resuscitation room. If there is a deterioration in any of these parameters, hypoxia or hypotension must be ruled out before considering an intracranial injury.

The *consciousness level* is measured by using the Glasgow Coma Scale (Figure 3). This records the best motor (Figures 4–9), verbal and eye opening responses to standard stimuli (Figures 10 and 11).

The *pupillary response* to a light stimulus is measured (Figure 12) and scored on the Glasgow Coma Scale (see Figure 3).

Lateralizing signs detect asymmetry of motor response. A sensitive test for partial hemiplegia in the conscious patient is to monitor the upper limb drift, the earliest sign being pronation of the palm (Figure 13).

Base of skull
Fractures to the base of the skull produce signs along a diagonal line extending from the mastoid process to the eye (Figure 14).

Bruising over the mastoid process (Battle's sign) and orbit can take 12–24 h to develop (Figures 15 and 16).

If there is no breach to the tympanic membrane, a haemotympanum may be detected on auroscopic examination of the ear. Cerebrospinal fluid rhino- and otorrhoea is invariably mixed with blood (Figure 17). This produces a double-ring pattern when some of the fluid is dropped onto an absorbent sheet. Another

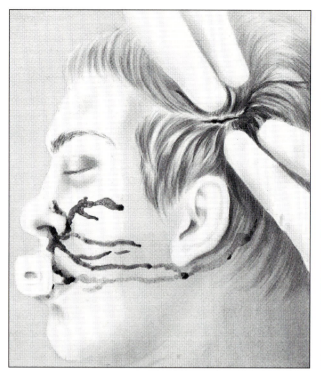

Figure 1 The whole scalp needs to be examined for lacerations, swellings or depressions

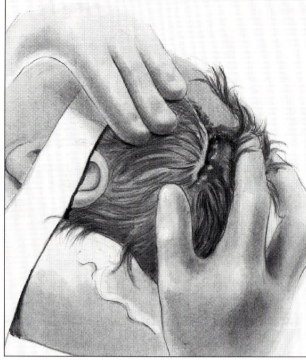

Figure 2 A close-up of a scalp laceration with a contusion revealed by retracting the hair

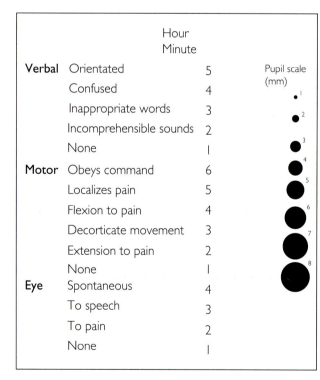

Figure 3 The Glasgow Coma Scale

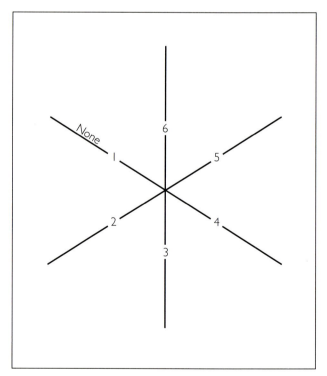

Figure 4 Glasgow Coma Scale, motor response

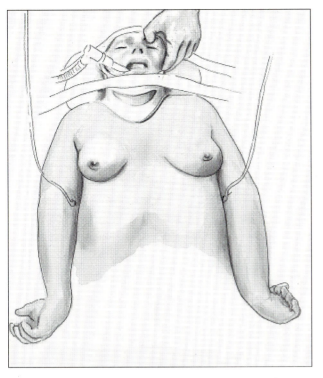

Figure 5 Motor response, score 2: extension to pain

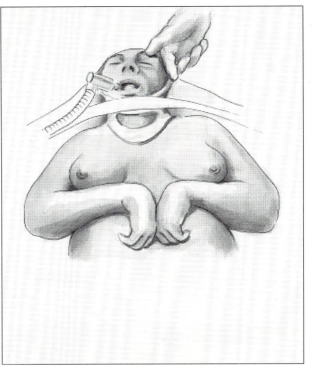

Figure 6 Motor response, score 3: decorticate movement

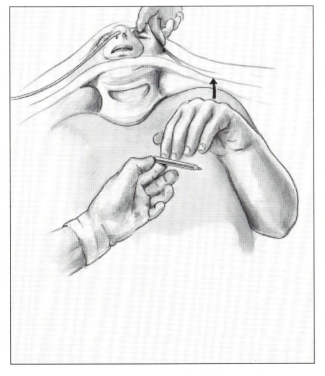

Figure 7 Motor response, score 4: flexion to pain

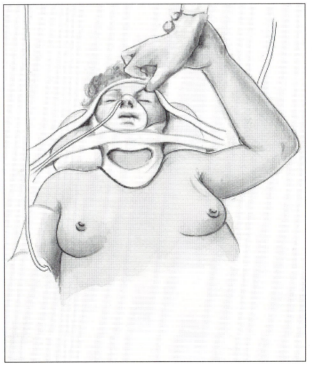

Figure 8 Motor response, score 5: localizes pain

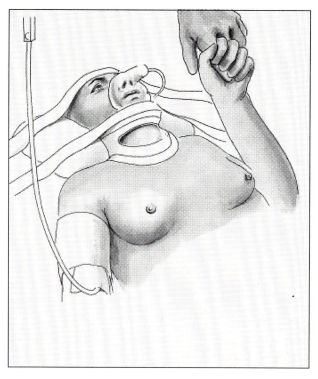

Figure 9 Motor response, score 6: obeys commands

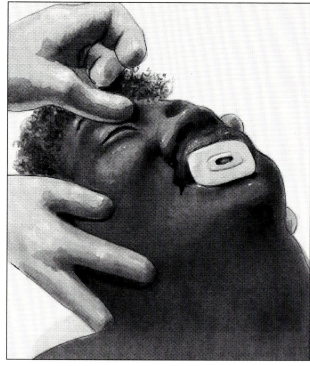

Figure 10 A painful stimulus, such as supratrochlear pressure

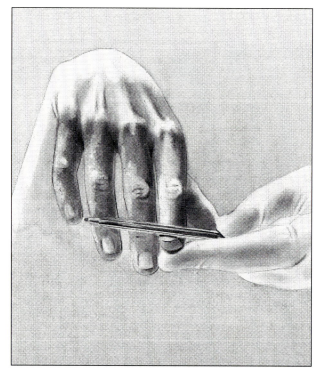

Figure 11 Another painful stimulus, pressure on the nail beds

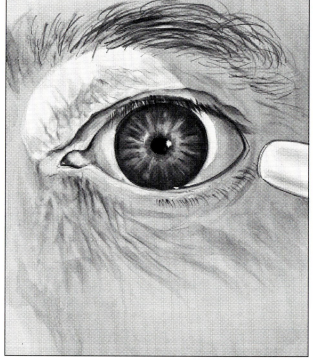

Figure 12 Measurement of response to light stimulus

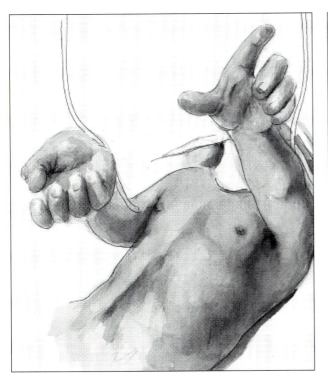

Figure 13 Pronation of the palm, a lateralizing sign

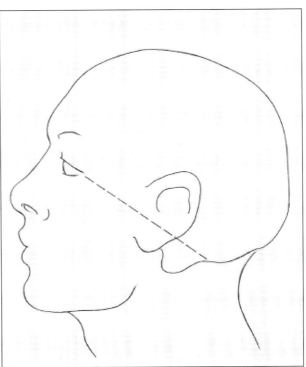

Figure 14 Fractures to the skull produce signs along a diagonal extending from the eye to the mastoid process

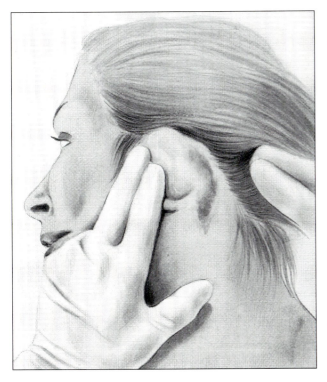

Figure 15 Bruising over the mastoid process – Battle's sign

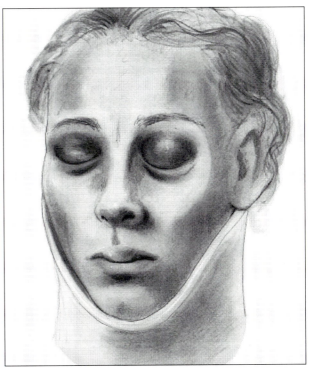

Figure 16 'Panda' eyes

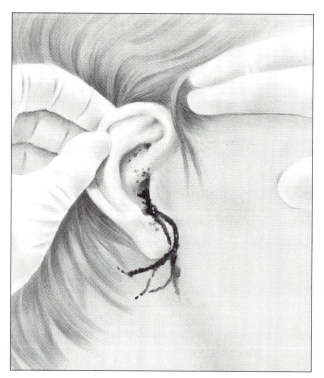

Figure 17 Cerebrospinal fluid otorrhoea

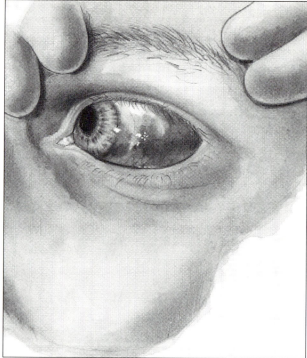

Figure 18 Scleral haemorrhage without a posterior margin

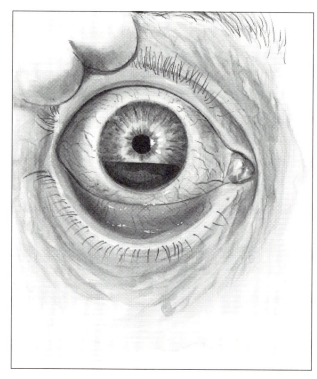

Figure 19 Hyphaema of the eye

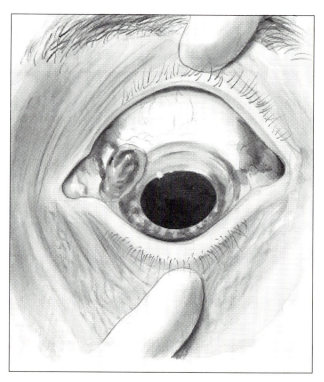

Figure 20 Herniating iris

method is to note the delay in clotting of the liquid running from the nose and ear. A leak of cerebrospinal fluid means that there is a compound fracture of the base of the skull and that the dura is torn. Many centres will treat these patients with antibiotics, but the local policy must be known by the attending clinician.

A nasogastric tube should not be inserted if a fracture at the base of the skull is suspected because there is a chance it may be pushed into the cranial vault. The tube should, therefore, be passed orally.

Scleral haemorrhages without posterior margins and subhyloid haemorrhages are also indicative of a fracture at the base of the skull (Figure 18).

Eyes

The clinician must inspect the whole of the eye for haemorrhages, foreign bodies and the presence of penetrating injury (Figures 19 and 20). If the patient is conscious, the visual acuity can be tested by having him/her read a label on the fluid bottle. If they are unconscious, the pupillary response and corneal reflexes are assessed (Figure 21).

Face

The whole of the face has to be inspected for bruising and deformity (Figure 22). Simultaneous, symmetrical palpation of the bony margins helps the clinician to detect any step-off deformity, crepitus or tenderness.

Each side of the maxilla can then be pulled forward (Figure 23) to check for movement and assessment of a Le Fort fracture (Figures 24–27).

Middle third fractures are often associated with basal skull fractures. However, only those producing obstruction of the airway need to be treated immediately.

The malars (zygomas) must also be palpated in the same symmetrical manner (Figure 28).

The bridge of the nose is palpated (Figure 29) and each nostril inspected for septal haematoma and blood (Figure 30).

The mouth is then assessed for soft tissue trauma, loose or lost teeth and the stability of the mandible (Figures 31 and 32). Mandibular fractures can cause airway obstruction because of the loss of tongue stability. In these cases, the jaw thrust manoeuvre must be maintained.

Neck

All of the neck needs to be carefully examined. Therefore, the collar, sandbags and tape will have to be temporarily removed. During this time, an assistant must maintain manual in-line stabilization (Figure 33).

The neck is initially re-inspected for any distended neck veins, marks and wounds. The tracheal position is rechecked and then the whole of the neck palpated (Figure 34). Each spinous process is tested for tenderness or deformity. Both trapezius and sternomastoid muscles are also assessed for spasm and tenderness. Lacerations deep to the platysma should *not* be probed as this may precipitate a major haemorrhage. Further exploration should be carried out in an operating theatre.

Upon completion of the neck examination, the semi-rigid collar, sandbags and tape are replaced.

All victims of blunt trauma or injury above the level of the clavicles require a lateral cervical radiograph initially. A complete cervical series should be carried out during the definitive phase of the initial assessment.

THORAX

The presence of six potentially life-threatening thoracic conditions and three minor ones must be

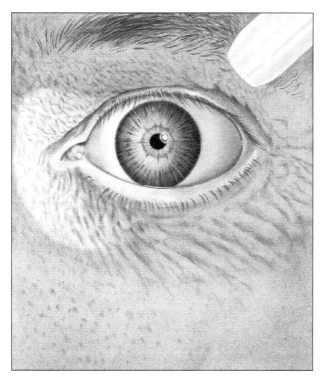

Figure 21 Pupillary response to light

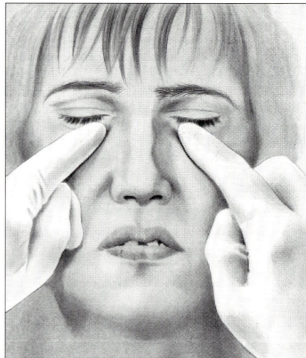

Figure 22 Inspection of face for bruising and deformity

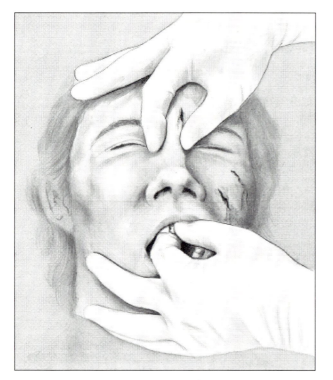

Figure 23 Testing for a Le Fort fracture

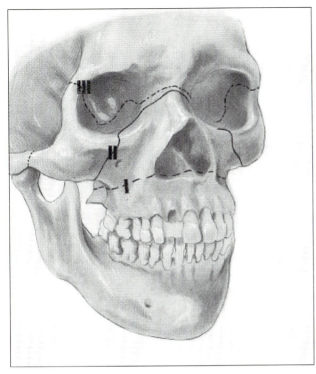

Figure 24 The Le Fort fracture lines

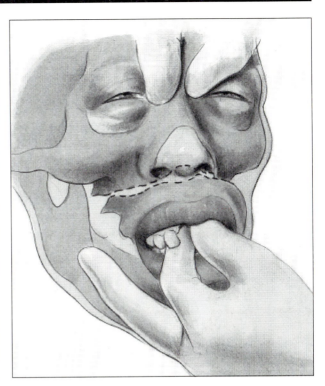

Figure 25 Le Fort I fracture line

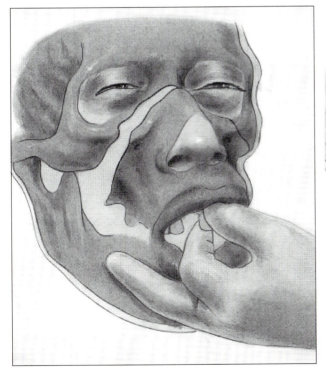

Figure 26 Le Fort II fracture line

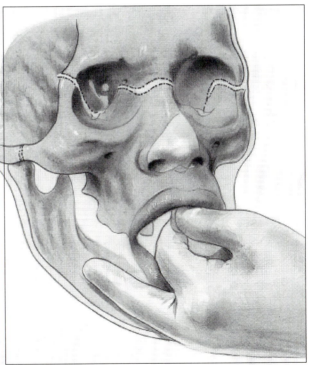

Figure 27 Le Fort III fracture line

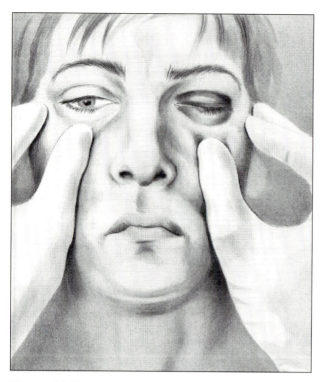

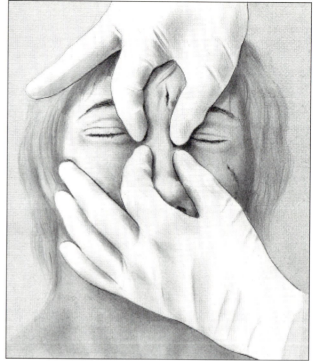

Figure 28 Palpation of the malars in a symmetrical manner

Figure 29 Palpation of the bridge of the nose

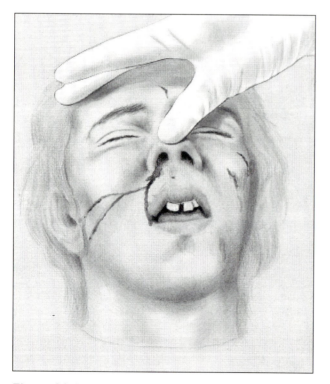

Figure 30 Inspection of nostrils for septal haematoma and blood

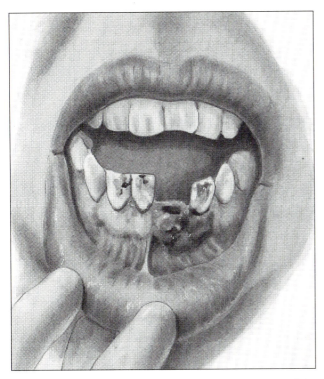

Figure 31 The inside of the mouth with haematoma of the lower gums and lost teeth with associated bleeding sockets

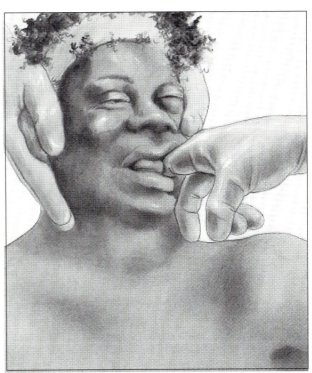

Figure 32 Assessment of mouth for soft tissue trauma, loose or broken teeth, and stability of the mandible

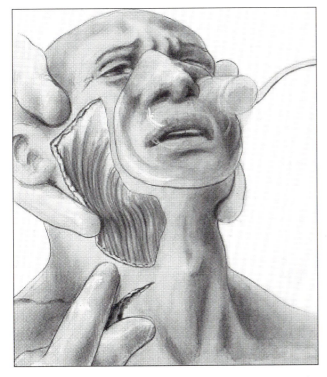

Figure 33 Careful neck inspection, lacerations deep to the platysma should not be probed

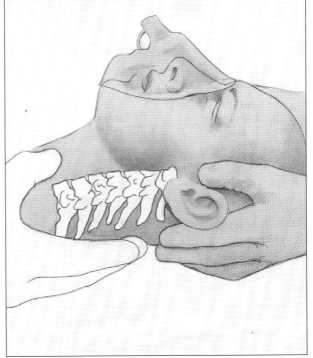

Figure 34 Palpation of the cervical vertebrae

detected in the secondary survey. The potentially life-threatening thoracic conditions are:

(1) Pulmonary contusion (Figure 35);

(2) Cardiac contusion (Figure 36);

(3) Ruptured diaphragm (Figure 37);

(4) Dissecting thoracic aorta (Figure 38);

(5) Oesophageal rupture (Figure 39);

(6) Airway rupture (Figure 39).

The three minor conditions are simple pneumothorax; haemothorax; and fractured ribs (Figure 40).

A thorough examination of the chest is therefore required. This is carried out by inspection, palpation, percussion and auscultation. In a similar way to the primary survey, the chest wall must be inspected for respiratory rate, symmetry of movement, marks and penetrating wounds (Figure 41).

Palpation of the whole chest (Figure 42) is carried out by feeling each rib in turn, starting in the apices of both axillae and continuing in a caudal manner. This is repeated over the anterior aspect of the chest from the clavicles to the costal margins (Figure 43). Any crepitus, surgical emphysema (Figure 44) or tenderness should be noted. The chest can then be squeezed in the lateral and anterior-posterior plane to detect the presence of multiple rib fractures (Figure 45). Auscultation and percussion of the chest are then carried out (Figure 46).

Pulmonary contusion
Pulmonary contusion is caused usually by a blunt injury transmitting its energy to the underlying lung tissue (Figure 47). There are often tenderness and marks over the chest wall due to causative impact. Overlying ribs may not be fractured in the young, because of the natural elasticity of the chest wall. Auscultation can also be normal initially. As the interstitial and alveolar

oedema develops, the patient develops respiratory distress (Figure 48).

A plain chest radiograph and arterial blood sample are essential (Figure 49).

Patients with this condition require a high forced expiratory oxygen, careful fluid administration and close observation in a high dependency unit. Many will go on to require sedation with pharmacological paralysis and positive pressure ventilation.

Cardiac contusion
Cardiac contusion should be suspected if the anterior chest has been subjected to a deceleration force, or if there is sternal bruising and tenderness (Figure 50). An ECG should be taken as this can reveal acute myocardial ischaemic changes and dysrhythmias, such as premature ectopic ventricular and atrial beats, bundle branch block and atrial fibrillation. This condition requires high dependency monitoring with standard treatment for the dysrhythmias.

Ruptured diaphragm
A ruptured diaphragm can follow either blunt or penetrating trauma (Figure 51). It should be suspected if there is trauma to the lower ribs or a penetrating wound between the 5th and 12th ribs. Breath sounds may be decreased over the affected area, but usually there are few physical signs.

Once the spine has been cleared radiologically and clinically, an erect chest X-ray may show an elevated hemidiaphragm, bowel herniating into the pleural space or the tip of a nasogastric tube above the diaphragm in the chest (Figure 52). This condition requires operative repair and surgical advice to rule out associated thoracic or abdominal injuries.

Dissecting thoracic aorta
Dissecting thoracic aorta occurs when the patient has been subjected to a rapid deceleration. A variety of signs may be present, such as hoarseness (Figure 53),

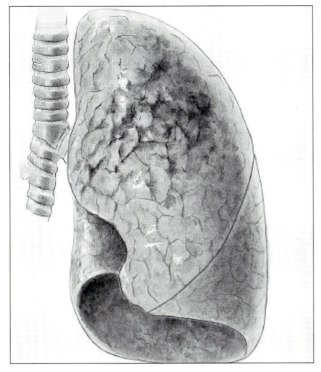

Figure 35 Pulmonary contusion

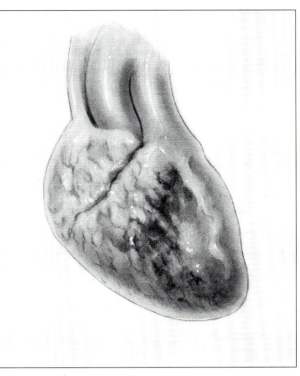

Figure 36 Cardiac contusion

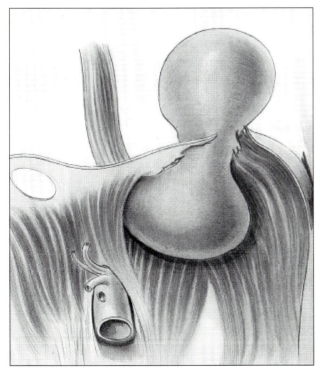

Figure 37 Ruptured diaphragm

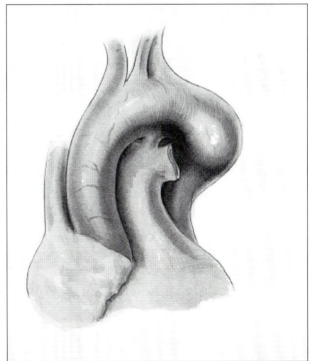

Figure 38 Dissecting thoracic aorta

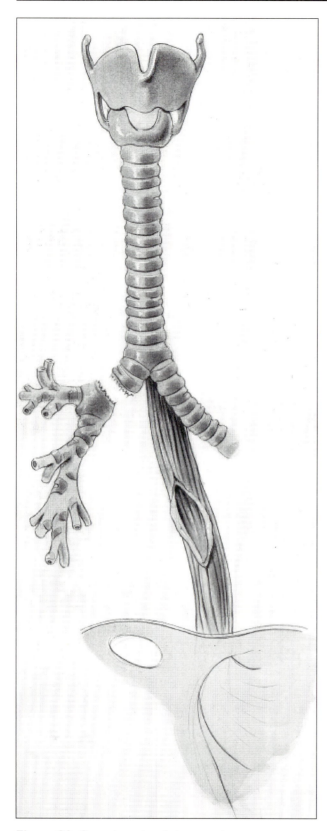

Figure 39 Oesophageal and airway ruptures

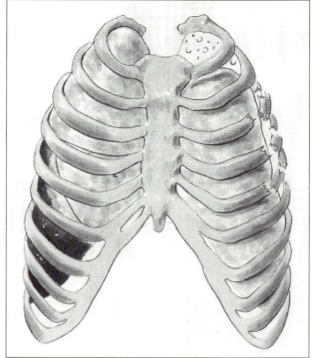

Figure 40 Three minor conditions – small haemothorax, simple pneumothorax and fractured ribs

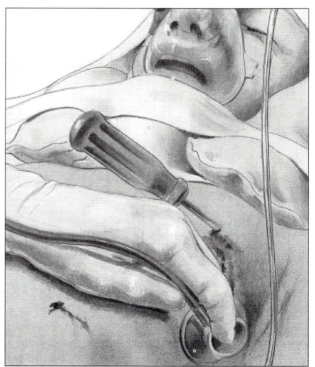

Figure 41 A penetrating wound

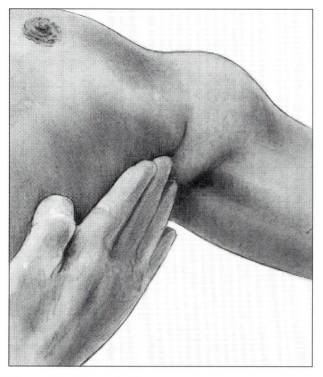

Figure 42 Chest palpation

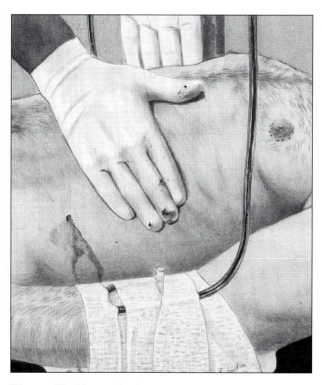

Figure 43 Chest palpation down to the costal margins

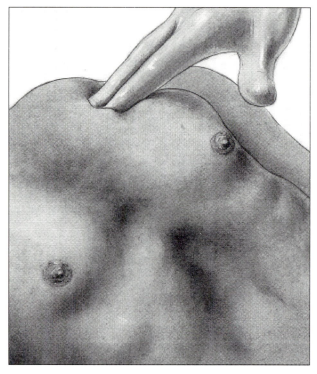

Figure 44 Surgical emphysema should be noted

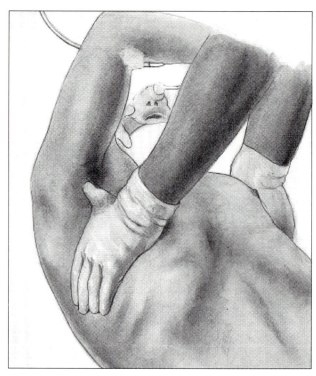

Figure 45 Lateral squeeze in chest palpation procedure

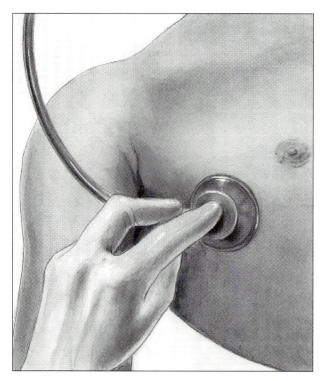

Figure 46 Auscultation of the axillae

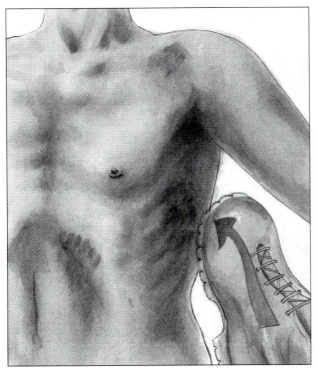

Figure 47 Blunt injury transmitting its energy to the underlying lung tissue

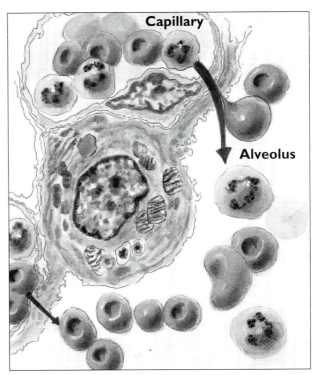

Figure 48 Interstitial and alveolar oedema

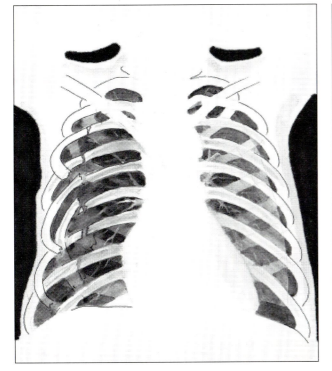

Figure 49 Lung contusion under a flail segment and also a contralateral pneumothorax, on a chest radiograph

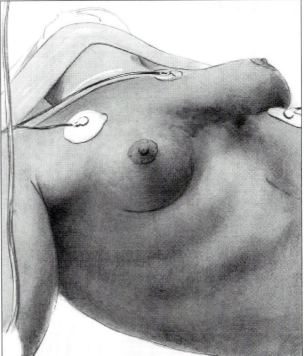

Figure 50 Signs of deceleration force and sternal bruising

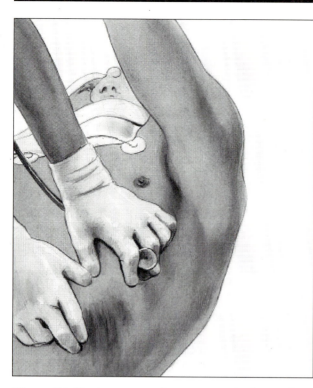

Figure 51 Blunt or penetrating trauma to the lower ribs

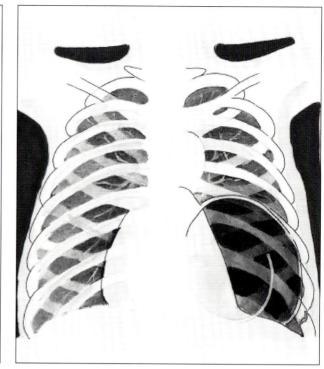

Figure 52 Radiological signs of a ruptured diaphragm

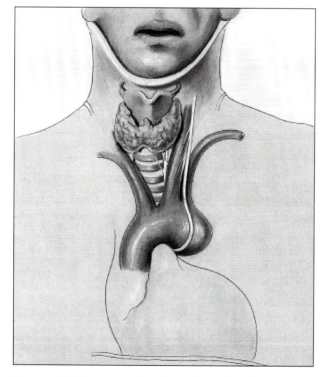

Figure 53 Hoarseness is a sign in dissecting thoracic aorta due to involvement of the recurrent laryngeal nerve

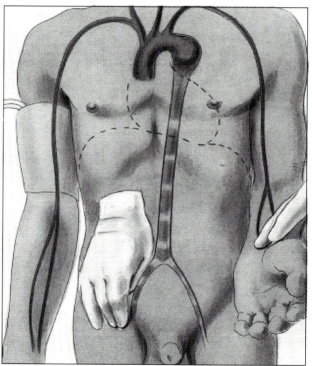

Figure 54 Upper limb hypertension and pulse pressure differences between the upper and lower limbs

upper limb hypertension and pulse pressure differences between the upper and lower limbs (Figure 54).

An erect chest X-ray is essential. A widened mediastinum is the most important sign but other features may be present (Figure 55), these being widened mediastinum, pleural capping, trachea deviated to the right, oesophagus deviated to the right, blurring of aortic notch, left mainstem bronchus depressed, right mainstem bronchus elevated, decrease in space between the pulmonary artery and aorta, and first and second rib fractures. These patients require urgent angiography of the aortic arch and surgery.

Oesophageal rupture

Oesophageal rupture can follow a penetrating injury at any level of the neck or thorax, or a severe blow to the epigastrium (Figure 56). The patient usually has a degree of shock and pain which is much greater than the apparent physical signs. Suspicion should be further raised if there is a left-sided pneumothorax without a history of left-sided trauma or fractured ribs (Figure 57). If an underwater chest drain has been inserted for the pneumothorax, the fluid level will swing during both expiration *and* inspiration. On the chest radiograph, a pneumomediastinum or a fluid level may be present behind the heart shadow (Figure 58). This condition requires further investigation and, in almost all cases, a surgical repair.

Airway rupture

This can occur at the larynx, trachea or bronchi and can follow either blunt or penetrating trauma (Figures 59 and 60).

These patients can present with a partial or complete obstruction of the airway, haemoptysis and neck wounds, swellings and marks (Figures 61 and 62). The first priority is to ensure that these patients have a patent airway. This may be technically difficult, so skilled ENT or anaesthetic advice should be sought early on.

All traumatic pneumothoraces are associated with some bleeding into the pleural space. As the bleeding usually stops spontaneously, the only treatment required is drainage of the blood and air through a large chest drain.

ABDOMEN

The abdomen should be first inspected for bruising, movement and wounds (Figure 63). Exposed bowel should be covered with a saline soaked swab. A systematic palpation should then be carried out, to detect signs of tenderness and guarding (Figure 64).

The management of stab wounds which penetrate muscle will depend on the state of the patient and the local policy. This should be known by the examining clinician.

The pelvis can also be squeezed laterally and over the pubis (Figure 65). However, these tests will only detect gross pelvic disruption. All patients with blunt abdominal trauma require a pelvic X-ray.

Urethral damage, in the male, should be suspected if there is blood at the end of the urethral meatus (Figure 66), bruising of the scrotum (Figure 67) and a high-riding prostate (Figure 68) on rectal examination. Percussion and auscultation of the abdomen can then be carried out (Figure 69).

A perineal examination and rectal examination should always be carried out during the secondary survey (Figure 70). The latter provides five pieces of information:

(1) Sphincter tone (Figure 71);

(2) Direct rectal trauma (Figure 72);

(3) Pelvic fractures (Figure 73);

(4) Prostate position (Figure 74);

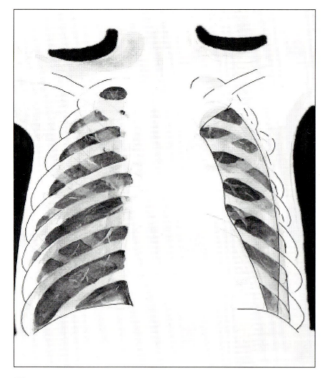

Figure 55 Radiological signs of dissecting thoracic aorta

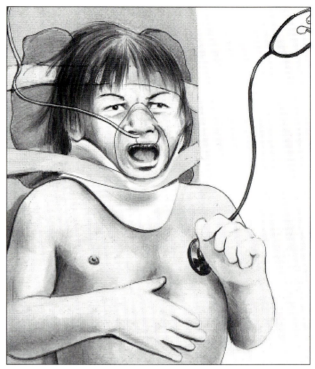

Figure 56 Oesophageal rupture causes a degree of shock or pain which is much greater than the apparent physical signs

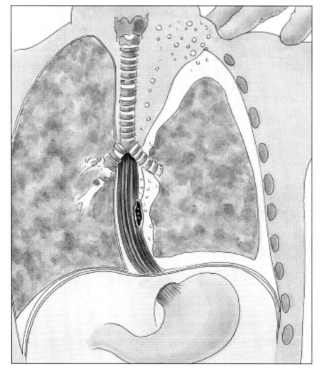

Figure 57 Signs of oesophageal rupture

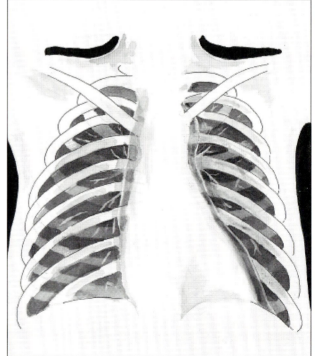

Figure 58 Radiological signs of oesophageal rupture

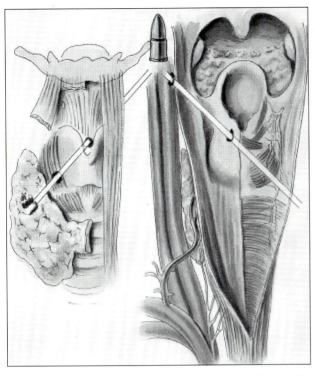

Figure 59 Damage to trachea and larynx caused by a bullet

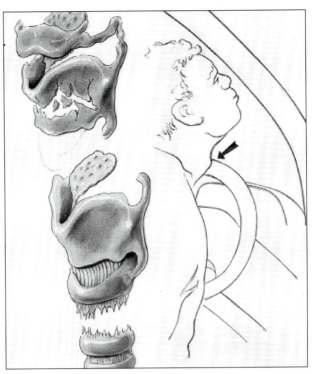

Figure 60 Damage to trachea and larynx caused by the neck hitting a dashboard. The larynx and trachea are compressed between the impacting object and the vertebral bodies

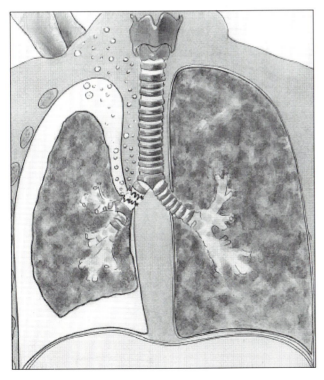

Figure 61 Signs of airway rupture

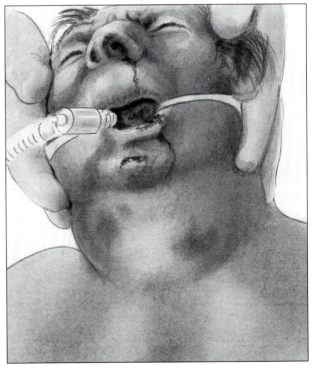

Figure 62 Signs of airway rupture include partial/complete obstruction of the airway, haemoptysis and neck wound

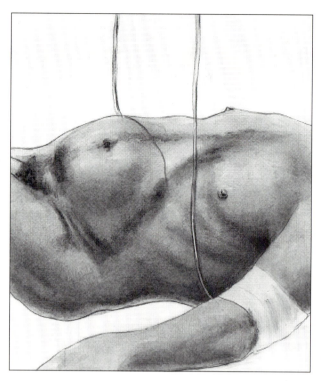

Figure 63 Abdomen showing marks and contusion

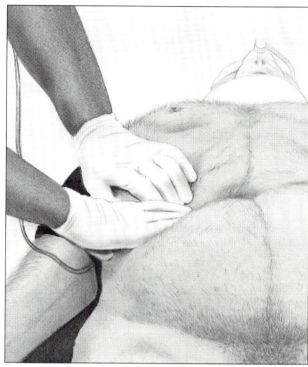

Figure 64 Systematic palpation to detect tenderness and guarding

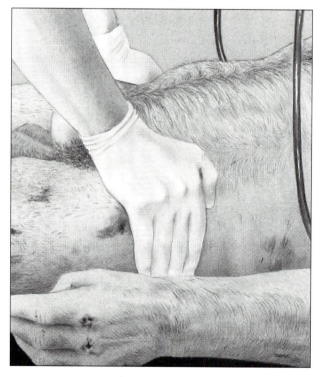

Figure 65 The pelvis can be squeezed laterally

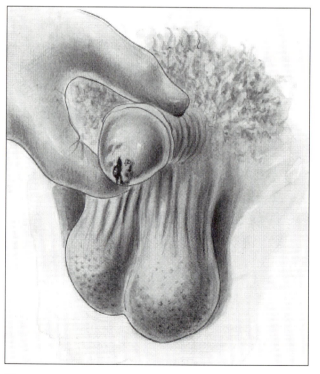

Figure 66 Blood at tip of the urethral meatus

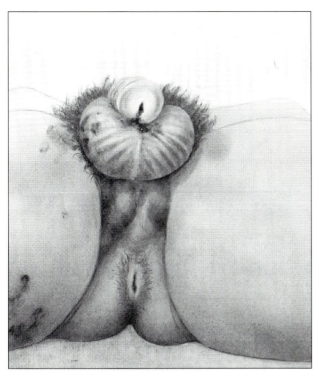

Figure 67 Bruising of scrotum

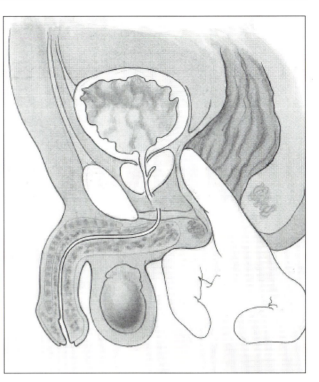

Figure 68 A high-riding prostate

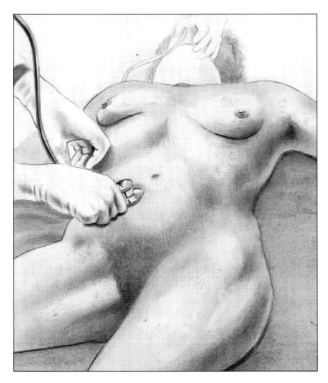

Figure 69 Auscultation of the abdomen

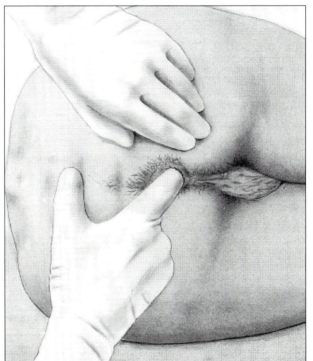

Figure 70 Rectal examination

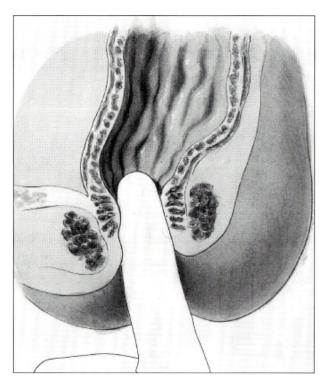

Figure 71 Sphincter tone

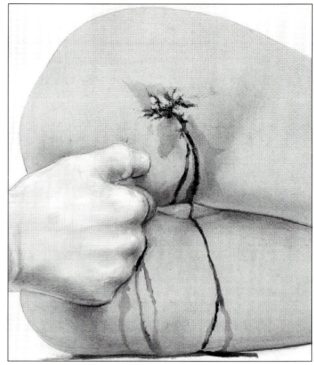

Figure 72 Direct rectal trauma

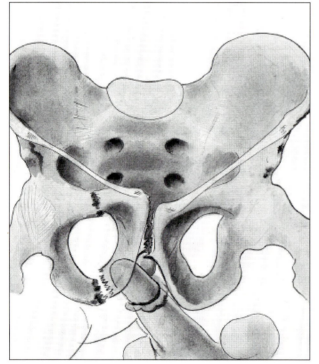

Figure 73 Pelvic fractures

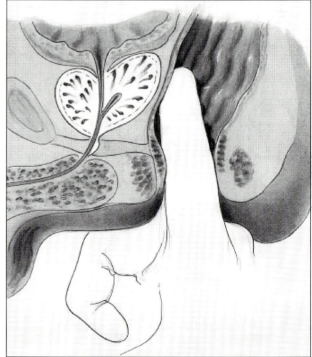

Figure 74 Prostate position

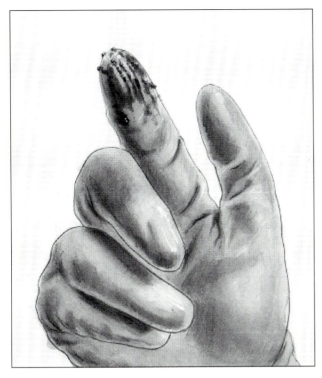

Figure 75 Blood in faecal residue

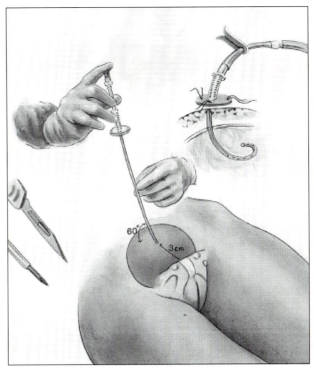

Figure 76 Procedure for insertion of suprapubic catheter

(5) Blood from the lower gastrointestinal tract in the faecal residue on the glove (Figure 75).

If there is no evidence of urethral damage, the urinary catheter can be inserted perurethrally. As described previously, this gives invaluable information on the adequacy of the fluid resuscitation. If the urethra has been damaged, a suprapubic catheter should be used instead (Figure 76). These patients will subsequently require a retrograde urethrogram.

The urine should be tested for blood. If it is positive, a one-shot intravenous pyelogram can be taken in the resuscitation room. This will show if both kidneys are present and functioning. This rapid investigation is usually only carried out in those patients requiring an urgent operation where the presence of any major renal pathology needs to be ruled out.

A gastric tube facilitates abdominal examination in those patients with marked gastric distension (Figure 77). This occurs more commonly in crying children, patients who have been ventilated with a bag and mask, and adults with head or abdominal injuries (Figure 78).

Intra-abdominal bleeding should be suspected if there are fractures to the ribs overlying the liver and spleen (ribs 5–11) (Figure 79), the patient is haemodynamically unstable, or if there are seatbelt and tyre marks over the abdomen. The detection of abdominal tenderness becomes unreliable if the patient has a sensory defect from neurological damage or drugs. In these cases a diagnostic peritoneal lavage should be performed to help rule out an intraperitoneal injury (Figures 80–84).

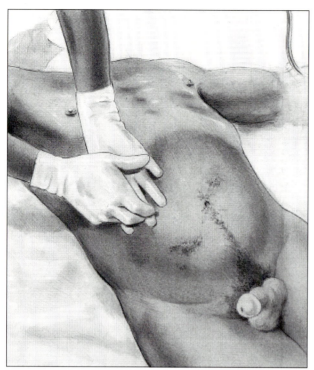

Figure 77 Marked gastric distension

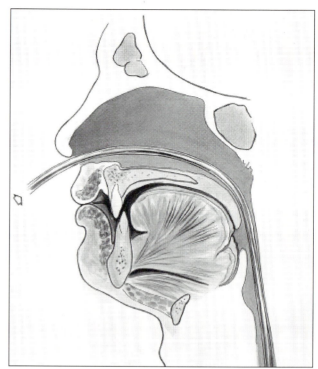

Figure 78 Procedure for insertion of nasogastric tube

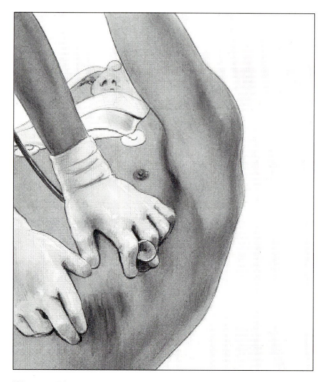

Figure 79 Intra-abdominal bleeding should be suspected if there are fractures to ribs 5–11 overlying the liver and spleen

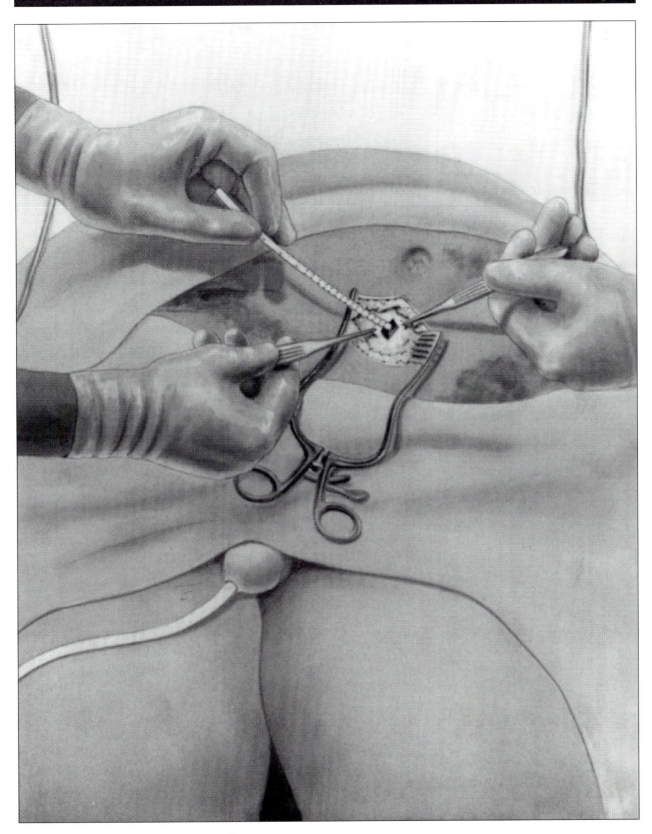

Figure 80 Diagnostic peritoneal lavage in progress on an abdomen showing marks and contusions

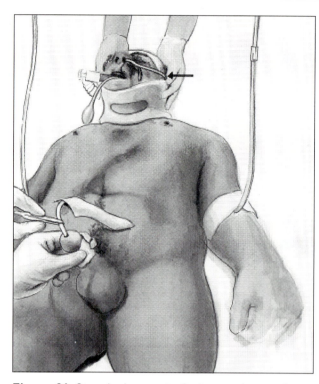

Figure 81 Stage I: placement of urinary catheter prior to peritoneal lavage, with the nasogastric tube already *in situ*

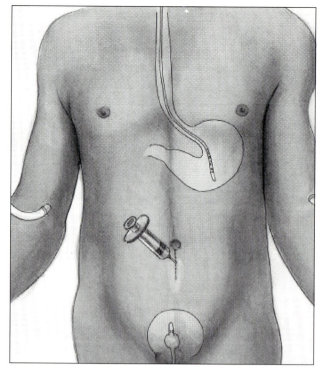

Figure 82 Stage II: infiltration with local anaesthetic, with the nasogastric tube and urethral catheter *in situ*

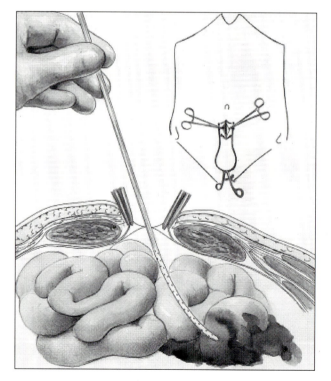

Figure 83 Stage III: introduction of cannula

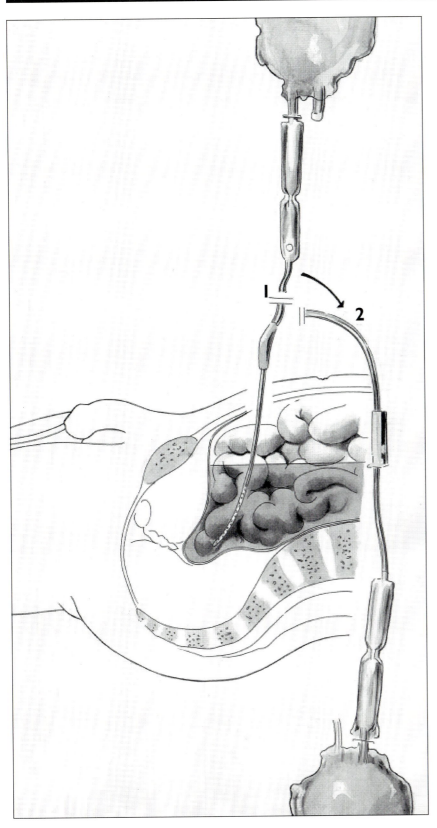

Figure 84 Stage IV: peritoneal lavage

EXTREMITY TRAUMA

The objective during this part of the secondary survey is to detect any limb-threatening condition and then find any other minor injuries.

Limb-threatening conditions are injuries which can result in the loss of function of all or part of a limb. These are:

(1) A vascular injury proximal to the elbow or knee (Figure 85);

(2) A major joint dislocation (Figure 86);

(3) Fracture with a major nerve injury (Figure 87);

(4) An open fracture (Figure 88);

(5) A crush injury (Figure 89);

(6) Compartment syndrome;

(7) Amputation (Figure 90).

The limbs are examined using a 'look, feel and move' technique.

Look

A thorough inspection of all the extremities must be carried out (Figure 88). Any swellings, deformities, bruising, wounds and marks should be noted. Shortening or rotation usually indicates there is a proximal fracture or dislocation. The viability of skin overlying the fracture or deformity must be checked.

Feel

The limbs should then be felt to assess the presence of tenderness, crepitus, altered sensation or vascular impairment (Figure 91). Signs of vascular impairment are skin pallor, cold skin, pain – increasing with passive movement (compartment syndrome), paraesthesia, paralysis, and distal pulse impairment. A diminished pulse should be assumed to be due to vascular injury until this has been excluded by further investigations. The clinician should never assume a weak pulse is simply due to vascular spasm. Doppler devices can be used to help detect distal circulation (Figure 92). Third-degree circumferential burns may impede distal circulation and so prompt escharotomy (Figure 93).

Move

If the patient is conscious, he/she should be asked to move each limb in turn (Figure 94). The extremities can then be passively moved by the clinician. Any weakness and limitation in movement must be accurately noted.

Gross limb deformities can lead to significant soft tissue ischaemia and necrosis (Figure 95). They result from fractures or dislocations. When the covering tissue is severely compromised, these deformities need to be corrected, and pulses rechecked, before any radiographic investigation is carried out.

Compound fracture wounds should be photographed with a polaroid camera before being covered with a non-adherent dressing (Figure 96). The picture minimizes repeated explorations of the wound.

All limb fractures must be splinted to reduce fracture movement, and so reduce pain, bleeding, fat emboli formation and further soft tissue damage (Figure 97). After splintage the pulses and distal circulation must be re-assessed.

A compartment syndrome occurs when the pressure in the fascial compartment rises to a level higher than that in the supplying capillaries (Figure 98). This results from the limb muscles swelling following trauma. As the high pressure impedes their own blood perfusion, tissue ischaemia is produced. This condition should be suspected if there is (Figure 99):

(1) Increasing pain in the limb;

(2) Increasing pain on passive movement of the distal limb;

(3) A palpably tense compartment;

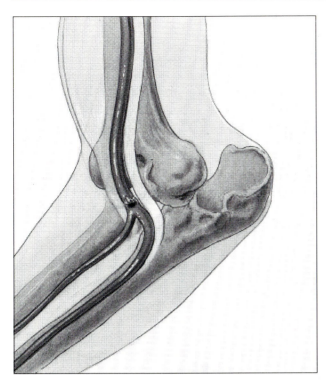

Figure 85 Vascular trauma proximal to elbow

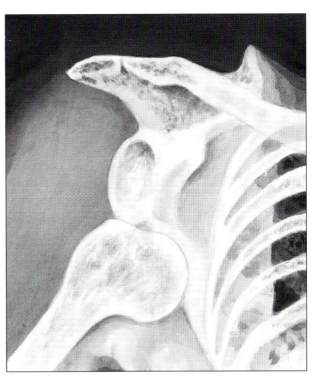

Figure 86 A major joint dislocation

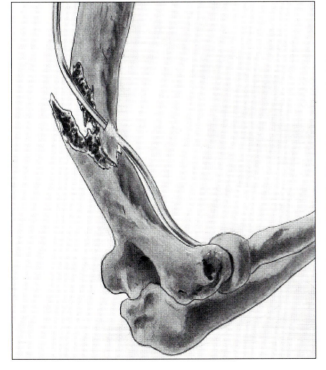

Figure 87 Fracture with a major nerve injury

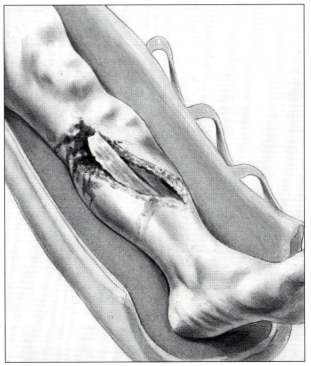

Figure 88 An open fracture of the tibia

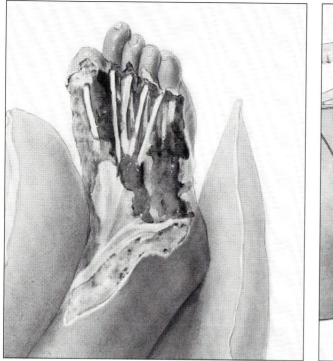

Figure 89 Crush injury

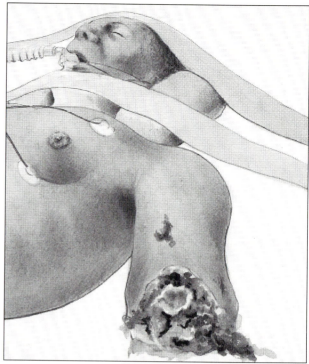

Figure 90 Amputation

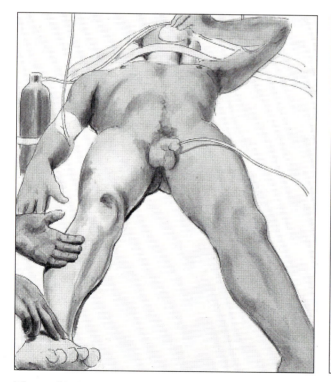

Figure 91 Signs of vascular impairment

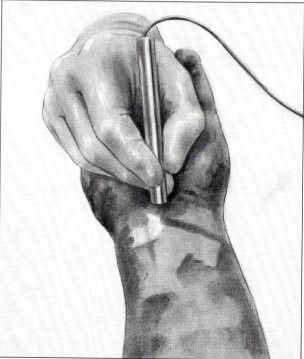

Figure 92 Doppler devices can be used to detect distal circulation

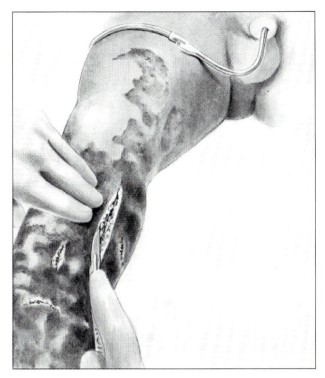

Figure 93 Escharotomy

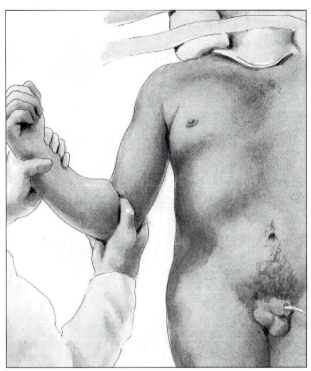

Figure 94 If the patient is conscious, he/she should be asked to move each limb in turn

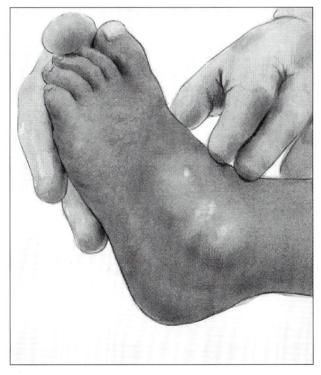

Figure 95 Gross limb deformities can lead to significant soft tissue ischaemia and necrosis

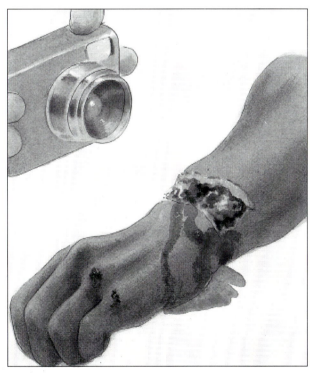

Figure 96 Compound fracture wounds should be photographed before being dressed

(4) Weakness of the affected muscles;

(5) A decrease in sensation of the nerves going through the compartment;

(6) Decrease in pulse pressure in the distal limb.

A decrease in pulse pressure in the distal limb is a *late* sign and indicates imminent tissue ischaemia.

This condition should be managed by removing all constricting clothing or splints. Usually this first-aid measure is inadequate and a fasciotomy is required.

Amputated limbs or digits remain viable for reimplantation for up to 18 h if wrapped in moist gauze, placed in a waterproof bag and covered with *melting ice* (Figure 100). Stumps of the amputated extremity should be covered with a pressure dressing.

Analgesia

Limb injuries are usually extremely painful. Consequently analgesia is required for both humanitarian and physiological reasons. Correct immobilization is extremely important in gaining pain relief. To help achieve this, Entonox, systemic analgesia or regional analgesia can be used (Figure 101).

SPINAL INJURIES

A detailed neurological examination of the whole of the patient is now required. The clinician should test for sensory and motor defects (Figures 102–113) and in the male patient, note any degree of priaprism.

Neurogenic shock will result if the cord is transected above the level of the sympathetic outflow (Figure 114). This takes the form of hypotension without any associated tachycardia.

The back is examined by turning the patient in a co-ordinated fashion, a manoeuvre known as a 'log-roll' (Figure 115). This requires at least five people. One must be at the 'head end' of the patient to support the neck whilst three others are positioned as indicated in the diagram. The clinician inspecting the patient makes up the fifth member of the team. All movement is under the command of the clinician stabilizing the cervical spine. It is essential that the turning action is carried out at the same rate and to the same extent by all team members. In this way, torsion of the vertebral column is avoided. The patient should also be asked to go 'stiff' or 'board like' prior to turning if he is conscious and co-operative.

The patient is turned away from the clinician so that the whole of the back is exposed. After inspection, the chest is auscultated and the occiput and vertebral column palpated. Any deformity, boggyness or tenderness must be noted. The patient is then 'log-rolled' back into the supine position.

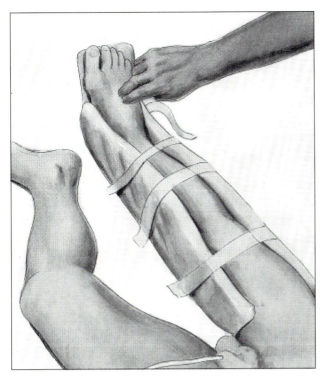

Figure 97 All limb fractures must be splinted

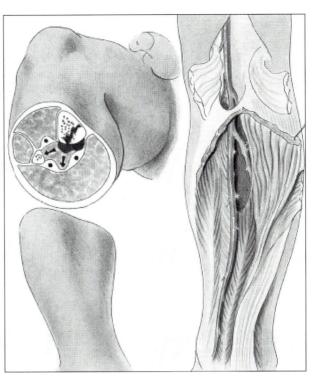

Figure 98 Compartment syndrome

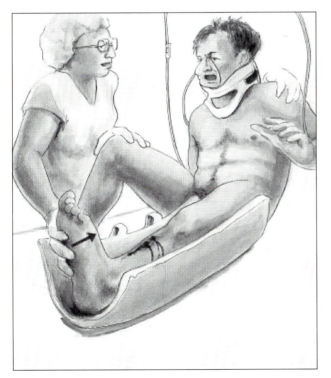

Figure 99 A sign of compartment syndrome

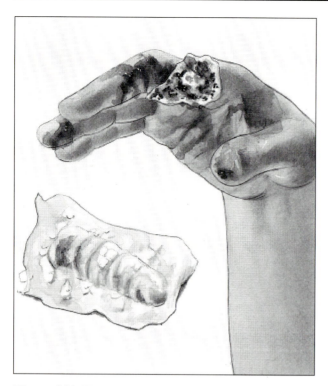

Figure 100 Treatment of amputated digit

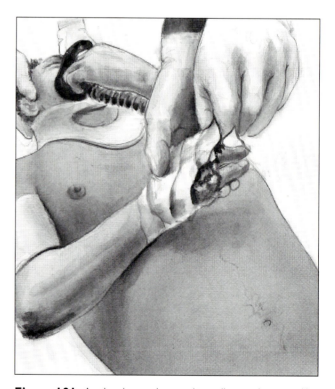

Figure 101 Analgesia may be used to relieve pain caused by limb injuries

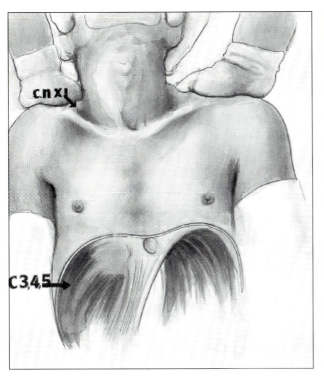

Figure 102 Test for defects in cranial nerve XI and C3, 4 and 5

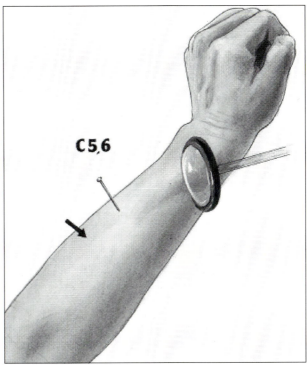

Figure 103 Test for defects in C5 and C6

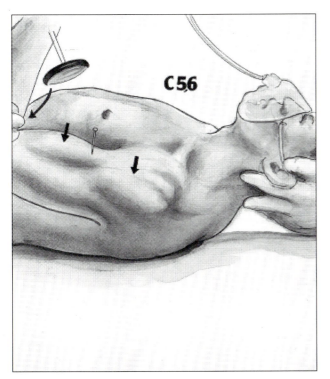

Figure 104 Test for defects in C5 and C6

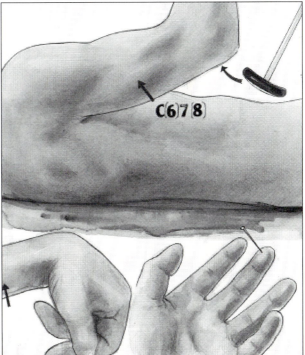

Figure 105 Test for defects in C6, 7 and 8

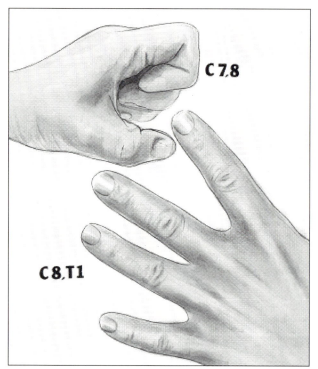

Figure 106 Test for defects in C7, C8 and T1

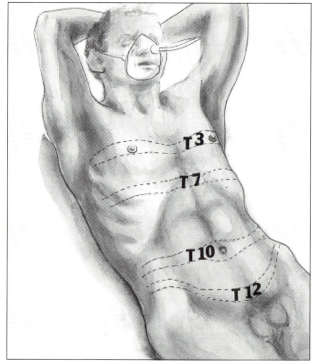

Figure 107 Test for defects in T3, 7, 10 and 12

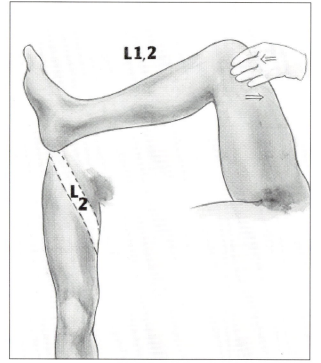

Figure 108 Test for defects in L1 and L2

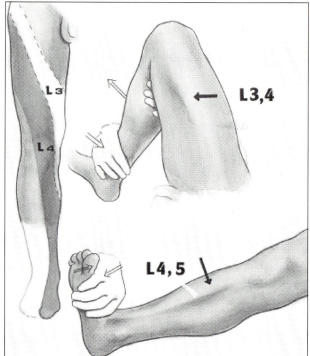

Figure 109 Test for defects in L3, 4 and 5

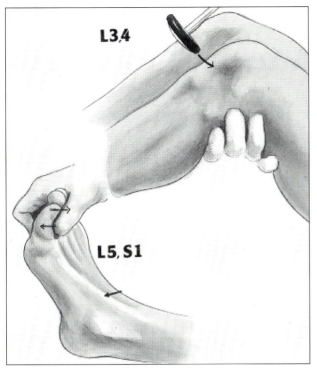

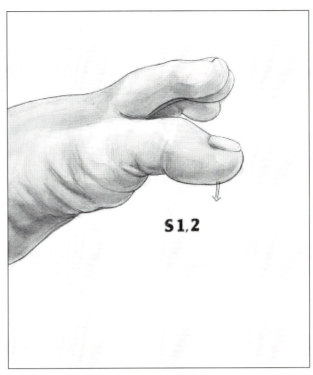

Figure 110 Reflex tests for defects in L3, 4 and 5, and S1

Figure 111 Sacral sparing in S1 and S2, shown by flexing of the big toe

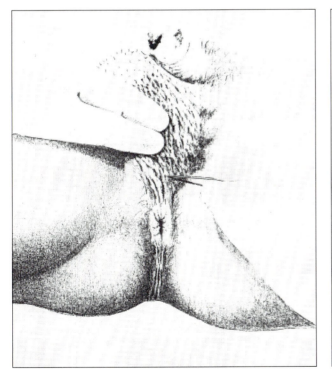

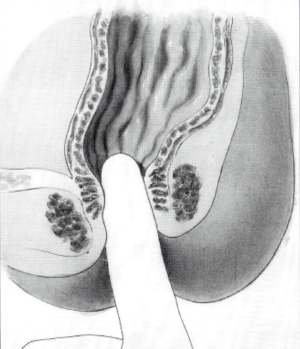

Figure 112 Test for sacral sparing

Figure 113 Assessment of sphincter tone

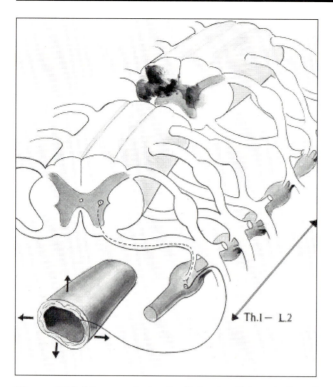

Figure 114 Neurogenic shock will develop if the spinal cord is transected above the level of the sympathetic outflow

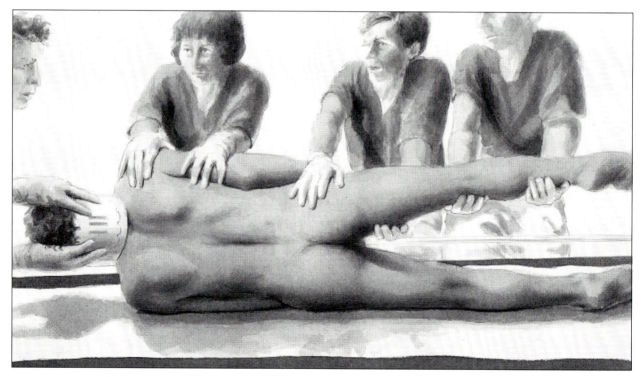

Figure 115 The 'log roll'

9

Stabilization and transfer

The definitive care of the patient takes place as soon as the patient has been assessed fully, resuscitated and three radiographs taken. Further delay in the Emergency department will frequently culminate in a deteriorating situation with an unclear diagnosis.

The management options of the team leader are:

(1) Immediate transfer to the operating department for definitive surgery;

(2) Transfer to the intensive care ward;

(3) Referral to a specialist centre;

(4) Specialized procedures in the radiology suite;

(5) Full radiological investigation, before transfer to the ward or home;

(6) Mortuary.

TRANSFER TO OPERATING THEATRE

The decision to operate should be made by the most senior person available, preferably the consultant in charge, as he or she carries the ultimate responsibility for management.

Failure to stabilize the haemodynamic state of the patient usually indicates that resuscitation should be continued in the operating room. Therein, full monitoring facilities are at hand and theatre staff can prepare for laparotomy or the application of an external fixator to the pelvis, as appropriate. Arteriograms, too, can readily be performed on the operating table.

TRANSFER TO INTENSIVE CARE

Intensive care, with ventilation and full monitoring, is suitable for the patient who requires ventilatory support. Other indications include severe head-injured patients not needing surgery and burn patients, with inhalational injuries. Frequent reassessment must be performed by the surgeon after transfer, as an operation could prove necessary at a later stage.

REFERRAL TO A SPECIALIST CENTRE

The treatment of trauma world-wide shows a considerable range of standards. Regional trauma units with full thoracic and neurosurgical expertise represent the 'state-of-the-art' units. These are widespread but still not universal in the USA. A lower provision is seen in most UK units, which have to maintain a high level of trauma management, with the sporadic arrival of a patient with multiple injuries and only distant specialist back-up.

A 'resuscitate and transfer' regimen may be the rule when the capabilities of the hospital are exceeded. The decision made by the team leader, in association with his consultant, concerning the disposal of the patient is on occasion extremely difficult. It must be emphasized that inappropriate movement for a neurosurgical opinion, in an inadequately resuscitated and stabilized patient, has led to many unnecessary deaths.

Indications for neurosurgical referral are:

(1) Abnormal computerized tomography scan;

(2) Skull fracture and neurological signs;

(3) Compound or depressed skull fracture;

(4) Base of skull fracture;

(5) Post-traumatic epilepsy;

(6) A deterioration in the neurological state;

(7) A Glasgow Coma Scale of 8 persisting after resuscitation;

(8) Amnesia of over 10 min;

(9) Neurological impairment persisting beyond 6–8 h even if there is no skull fracture.

Communication by the referring team leader should be on a one-to-one basis with the receiving physician. Adequate documentation should accompany the patient, including any radiographs taken. Details of treatments and fluid given should be unequivocal. Accurate notes are also of great importance retrospectively for audit and medicolegal work. They should be compiled as soon as is feasible with a clear entry from the team leader, signed, dated and the time recorded.

Preparation must be made for clinical deterioration during the journey. A sufficiently senior anaesthetist, versed in the monitoring and therapeutic equipment available, should escort the patient. The patient should be intubated and ventilated before transfer, if there is any likelihood that the airway requires protection. In addition to intubation, suction and intravenous cannulation instruments, adequate oxygen, blood and intravenous fluids are absolute requirements. A suitable ventilator, an ECG monitor, pulse oximeter, capnograph and infusion pump equipment are available on sophisticated ambulances. The transfer may be effected by ambulance or helicopter. Excessive braking or acceleration of either vehicle will cause detrimental cardiovascular changes. Furthermore, a Trendelenburg position is contraindicated in head injuries as it can lead to a rise in intracranial pressure.

SPECIALIZED RADIOLOGICAL PROCEDURES

Specialist radiological procedures may be sought prior to surgery or specialist referral. A computerized tomogram is particularly useful in diagnosing head injuries and defining surgically treatable conditions, for example intracranial haematoma from diffuse brain injury. It is also of great value in investigating spinal and acetabular fractures and can detect visceral and retroperitoneal haematomata.

Arch aortography is used to diagnose aortic rupture and arteriography to establish the arterial bleed amenable to embolization in fractures of the pelvis, or the extent of damage in a limb artery. The on-call radiologist will be required to perform and interpret these studies.

FULL RADIOLOGICAL INVESTIGATION

A stable patient can be transferred to the radiology suite for a skeletal survey for fractures and dislocations. A single-shot intravenous imaging of the renal tract may be indicated if haematuria is detected. Close observation of the patient's neurological and haemodynamic state should be continued by an accompanying nurse.

MORTUARY

A patient who is dead upon arrival or who perishes, despite resuscitative efforts, will need to be referred to the coroner's officer. Care must be taken of distressed relatives. If possible, a room should be made available.

Audit of the team's work should be an integral part of the conclusion of management. If time permits, a debriefing will highlight strengths and weaknesses. A formal monthly review of cases is of great educational value. Trauma-scoring systems taking physiological and/or anatomical parameters of the patient can be applied to predict the likelihood of survival.

10
Conclusion

The provision of optimal care for the patient with multiple injuries has been shown to reduce mortality rates substantially.

There is a strong case for a universal approach to these patients. It is essential that the chain of events extending from prehospital care to rehabilitation is maintained at a high standard. This is particularly true for the 'golden hour' of the patient's management, when poor decisions can lead to significant morbidity and mortality.

Index